ED.

(

IN SEARCH OF JERUSALEM

BOOKS BY MICHAEL KUSTOW

The Book of Us (John Calder, 1965)

Tank, An Autobiographical Fiction (Cape, 1975)

theatre@risk (Methuen, 2003)

Peter Brook, a Biography (Bloomsbury, 2005)

The Half: Actors Prepare for the Stage – text for Simon Annand's photographs (Faber, 2008)

IN SEARCH OF JERUSALEM

Michael Kustow

OBERON BOOKS

LONDON

First published in 2009 by Oberon Books Ltd
521 Caledonian Road, London N7 9RH
Tel: 020 7607 3637 / Fax: 020 7607 3629
e-mail: info@oberonbooks.com
www.oberonbooks.com

The photograph on page 49 is of a Lebanese victim of Israeli bombing, July 2006. (Wire service, source unknown.)

Cover image: portrait of Michael Kustow by Tom Phillips, 1987

ISBN: 978-1-84002-872-0

Printed in Great Britain by CPI Antony Rowe , Chippenham

To Bernard Kops

CONTENTS

AUTHOR'S NOTE

January 2009

This book is shadowed by wars. It began in the aftermath of Israel's bombardment of Lebanon in July 2006; it is being typeset two and a half years later, as Israel attempts to flush out Hamas, which continues sending rockets and terrorising the people of south Israel. The people of Gaza, who are killing no-one, are being indiscriminately slaughtered by the Israeli military.

For me, the two wars have been similar, but different. A model is being replayed at a perilous moment of the world. The Gaza war is similar to the Lebanese, in its initial, pulverising blitz; the asymmetry of a high-tech military machine against opponents living and fighting among the civilian population; the smokescreen of claims, counter-claims, threats and lies. In the heat of war, relentless TV coverage of carnage and wreckage rocks or emboldens one's opinions and shakes one's identity, if not one's convictions.

Gaza is different from Lebanon in one major fact: the Gazans have nowhere to flee. Gaza is a ghetto. The onslaught reminds me – and some Palestinians – of the decimation of the Warsaw Ghetto in World War Two. And it is a disproportionate response: in the words of historian Avi Shlaim, Israel's action and policy is 'an eye for an eyelash'.

You will not find anything about Gaza 2009 in the body of this book. The war is too volatile, I'm too close to see it clearly, yet I needed to make reference to it. The consequences of the Gaza conflict may be momentous. But in describing Lebanon 2006, I feel I'm expressing many aspects of an archetypal war and of one person's experience – a European and a troubled Jew – of the Middle East battle this year.

MK

I give you the end of a golden string
Only wind it into a ball
It will lead you in at Heaven's gate
Built in Jerusalem's Wall

William Blake, 'To the Christians' from *Jerusalem*

Like an army in the field which has to assure its supplies, they requisition adjoining blood vessels and force them to proliferate in order to provide oxygen and nutriments indispensable to the growth of what will rapidly become a tumour.

David Servan-Schreiber, *L'Anticancer*

I needed clarification, as much of it as I could get – demythologizing to induce depathologizing.

Philip Roth, *The Facts*

Do for Jews what Morandi did for Jars.

R B Kitaj (1932–2007), *Second Diasporist Manifesto*

SCENES FROM AN EARLIER LIFE

Scene 1: Opening Up

In gold letters on a black ground across the front of my father's shop in Tower Bridge Road, Bermondsey, it says A. KUSTOW AND SONS, CHILDREN'S OUTFITTERS.

My father opens up on a Saturday morning. Saturday for him means shop, not shul. *The shutters go up like a curtain rising. The windows are dressed with his hand-painted signs, done in black and red with a thick flat brush. I watched him every Wednesday night, window-dressing night. He made me unafraid of paint. He pinned wires lifting and spreading garments across the window-space, in frozen flight, executed with a care worthy of a great stage designer. He made the window his proscenium theatre.*

I went into the shop on Saturdays, to help him out. I would hang up strings of clothes outside the shop, reaching out to the passers-by, flaunting themselves into the street like a thrust stage under the shelter of our awning. I stood outside to shlep *the customers.* Shlep, *a Yiddish word meaning to pull them in.* Shlep. *Onomatopoeic, like so many Yiddish words –* shmuck, shemozzle, shyster, shtick. *When I came to Shakespeare I already knew about the meat of words, from Yiddish. 'Light thickens and the crow makes wing to the rooky wood.' Engliddish.*

'Come on in, my darlings, I've got something just for you! You should see our crazy prices! I need my head examined!' Glad I had that early

initiation into performance, those street theatre work-outs in Bermondsey more than half a century ago.

Scene 2: The chicken shed in the garden

I was the Gordon Craig, the Max Reinhardt of my home-made puppet-shows in that green chicken shed under the apple trees. I wrote, designed and performed the shows, and shlepped *in the punters from the houses along the street. I also did conjuring tricks. Hunted out manuals of magic in the children's library, made my props from their diagrams – metal rings, silk scarves, trick boxes, giant playing cards. When I performed at the Children's Library Christmas party, two little girls came round afterwards. 'We saw how you did it,' they said. 'You had a card hidden up your sleeve.' As it happens, for once I didn't. But I couldn't convince them.*

Artifice is a precious thing in the theatre. Audiences love to give in to the spell of artifice, and they also love to see through it. Theatre's essential doubleness.

Scene 3: Barmitzvah

I chanted my portion of the Torah on a raised platform in Golders Green Synagogue. It was called the bimah. *'What's a* bimah?' *my friends asked me. 'It's like an altar in church,' I said. I was only half right. I asked my friend Rami Elhanan from Jerusalem the root of the Hebrew word, and without hesitation he said, 'It means a stage.'* Bimah: *stage.* Ha-bimah, *the stage.*

Habimah is also the name of the first Hebrew actors' troupe in Russia, which was so good that Stanislavski and Vachtangov came to direct it, and Lunacharsky, Lenin's Minister of Culture, protected it from its many enemies, until he went down too. By the 1920s the future looked bleak for Habimah. They went on tour and did not return. Some of the company stayed in New York, where they influenced New York theatre, which, unlike British theatre, has always had a strong Russian/Jewish/Yiddish undercurrent. The rest of Habimah went to Palestine in 1927 and started to perform in Tel Aviv, which didn't even have a theatre building. Among their shows were the twin peaks of Yiddish theatre, Ansky's The Dybbuk *and Leivick's* The Golem. *That was Habimah, the Stage.*

And there I was in Golders Green Synagogue, a little boy standing on the bimah, *the altar, singing my heart out. I didn't just stand on it, I bestrode it. I had learned my Old Testament text by heart. Didn't understand every word, but loved the sound of the words, and the dots and squiggles underneath which were a vocal score. For the first time I had a dizzying sense of dominating the house, looking down on the heads of my elders, making my entrance into the fraternity of adults, at the tender age of thirteen.*

Houses of worship easily lend themselves to theatre. Years later, I went to see Arturo Ui *in the Half Moon Theatre in the converted synagogue in Alie Street, Whitechapel, where my father used to pray on High Holy Days, walking across Tower Bridge with his father to get there. You could still see the old stained-glass windows at the back of the stage. Brecht's pastiche Hitler on stage, and panes of coloured glass with Stars of David above him. Since then, I've seen plays in the crypts of churches, in quarries, in the gardens of a Buddhist retreat, in front of temples. Every time I go to Jerusalem, I want to do an Arab/Jewish/Christian play in the little squares of the Old City, in four languages – Arabic, English, Hebrew and the lost language of peace. Well, it's not forbidden to dream.*

Scene 4: Outdoors

The plays I saw in the college gardens of Oxford University lodge in memory. I vividly remember a production of Shakespeare's The Tempest *in a Worcester College garden at the edge of its lake. When Prospero gave Ariel his freedom, Ariel skated right across the surface of the water, scudding over the waves, and disappeared into the distant trees. Magic. Later I looked more closely, and of course there was a boardwalk just below the water surface.*

There's huge and sensuous expectation when you go to an open-air performance. It starts in daylight and you become aware that dusk is falling. The action advances as nature's light fades and stage light softly replaces it. You end up watching beneath the stars, as we did with John McGrath's production, in another college garden, of Aristophanes' The Birds. *It featured Dudley Moore as chorus leader, looking totally ridiculous in a bird-suit too big for him. Entering to George Shearing's* Lullaby of Birdland, *Dudley led a motley troupe of battered birds. At the end, they picked up instruments and became a storming band for the closing number, as fireworks flared above our heads.*

Theatre in Europe started on Greek hillsides under the sky. It went on all day in sunlight and finished when night fell. Tony Harrison, who has done more than anyone today to continue the totality of Greek theatre, calls the sun 'Nature's lighting rig'.

Scene 5: On the March

Still a student, I joined CND in 1960. I wanted to make theatre on the Aldermaston march. I'd found Out of the Flying Pan, *a trio of anti-war playlets by David Campton, and got Peggy Duff, the female Falstaff who led CND, to let us do them in the schools where marchers stayed overnight. We lashed up a stage among the Primus stoves and sleeping bags, magnified our performances to reach the corners of the hall, a bunch of fairground mountebanks using theatre of the absurd to expose nuclear lunacy.*

A couple of years later Peggy asked for a theatre piece in Trafalgar Square, at the end of the CND march. Adrian Mitchell wrote Punch and Judas, *an Aristophanic pageant for giant puppets. Gerald Scarfe painted cartoon faces of world leaders onto twenty-foot-high canvas flats on wheels; students manipulated the flats, actors at the side lent their voices to Harold Wilson, Ian Smith, LBJ. At the end we released hundreds of silver paper B-52s above the heads of the weary marchers, threw buckets of blood at the politicians' faces and watched the red paint dribble down as a folk singer sang Pete Seeger's* Turn Turn Turn, *lyrics from Ecclesiastes. Political theatre has to keep close to the street. I had discovered the link between* shlepping *customers in front of my dad's shop and punching home a message with the devices of circus, carnival and fiesta.*

Scene 6: Europe

In 1961 I left Oxford, not knowing what to do, or rather knowing there were too many things in Britain I didn't want to do, like joining the BBC, which many of my contemporaries were doing. I had a heavy sack filled with Jewish inheritance on my back and I needed to embrace it or exorcise it. I went to Israel and worked on a kibbutz, picking apples and collecting garbage, having Tolstoyan moments at dawn with the sun coming up, the grass dew-heavy and the cocks crowing.

But after three months I ran out of things to talk about with my peers. I could discuss Marxism with the Hungarian founders of the kibbutz, but they were old enough to be my parents; I had little common experience with the young men and women of my own age, athletic, taciturn, untravelled and army-trained.

I took a boat back to France, which, growing up on a diet of Baudelaire and Rimbaud and Artaud, I had elected in my imagination as my alternative homeland. I stopped in Lyon to see the work of Roger Planchon, whom I had read about in French theatre magazines. Planchon, then in his early twenties, was an incisive actor, compact and weighty yet light on his toes like Michael Gambon, and a brilliant director of the leading young company in the French théâtre populaire *movement.*

I saw his productions of Marlowe's Edward the Second *– brutal, poetic – and Marivaux's* La Seconde surprise de l'amour *– poignant,* *erotic – and I was hooked. I had to join this troupe somehow. This was my moment of running away to join the circus, of making the break with my origins, of striking out in a new language, a new land.*

I remember Planchon as a pile-driver of a man. Bunched muscle behind an intelligent head, eyes twinkling behind wire frames. Powerful torso, hands searching, legs elegant. Something feminine within his male force. A metallic voice. A crazed otherness in the world.

He saw himself as a peasant, from the dying region of the Ardèche. His father and mother, unable to make a living farming, came to Lyon, ran a café near the station. He was educated in a seminary by the Jesuits; a father caught him hopping over the wall to see an American movie in town. Instead of punishing Roger, he told him to go and see decent films – Bresson, Welles – and gave him, he told me, his first insight into quality. He went to work as a runner for the Westminster bank in Lyon. In the coffee bars of the early 'sixties, he watched poets reading their work, discovered poetry.

He met Isabelle Sadoyan, a seamstress; Jean Bouise, a gangling comic; and Colette Dompietrini, who became his wife. They watched movies to learn how to act. It was the heyday of the combative film magazine Cahiers du Cinéma, *from which they learned to revere Jerry Lewis as a master of* le gag. *They began performing plays in local halls. In an old print shop, he started a young company with his friends; Bouise, a carpenter, built the stage and auditorium. Roger devoured books like meals. He was fascinated by the German romantic poets Kleist and Lenz, with their madness, rebellion and search for new forms. From him I first learned the word* autodidacte, *self-taught. At first I thought it was some kind of illness; and perhaps it was, in a culture that so over-prized cleverness and intellectuality. He was seeking a different tradition outside the French consensus.*

Roger called his company the Théâtre de la Cité. *They found a home in Villeurbanne, a suburb half an hour from the centre of Lyon, and took over the old municipal theatre, between the police station and the town swimming pool. They polled local people, asking them what play they would like to see. There was an overwhelming vote for Alexandre Dumas'* Les Trois Mousquetaires, *so they did their version and kept updating, reviving and playing it for ten years. It became their economic banker, and theatrical test-bench. It was Dumas to a cha-cha beat, with Roger as a swashbuckling, self-mocking D'Artagnan. It was a youthful blitz on French conservatism, pop art theatre, an* hommage *to the American musical, a parody of current theatrical styles – Claudel, Brecht. When I joined the company, I swirled a banner in the production. I was too nervous to play the villainous Englishman le Duc de Buckingham, for which Roger auditioned me; my stammer got in the way. Roger directed the two parts of Shakespeare's* Henry IV *and played Prince Hal. They promoted the plays as* Un Grand Western Historique. *They publicised their theatre with lunchtime visits to factory canteens and group bookings organised with the trades unions.*

Later came the cruel comedy of his Molière productions, the rural realism of Georges Dandin, *the ferocious attack of his* Tartuffe. *The insolent resistance of his version of Brecht's* Schweik in the Second World War *mirrored the French* maquis *and the struggles around the Algerian war which in 1961 were tearing France apart. He was a* contestataire *long before 1968.*

Though his theatre was nominated and subsidised as a national company, le Théâtre National Populaire, *Roger came from outside the mainstream of French culture, and liked to talk about himself as 'un naïf.' He was the theatrical equivalent of Douanier Rousseau or Chagall, while at the same time learning directorial style from the masters of cinema, applying William Faulkner's time-shifts to his staging, and from Sartre learning political engagement and pessimism about human relationships.*

Depression lay behind his energy. He was obsessed by the history of suicide in his own family; it became the subject of his first play, La Remise. *He was a scathing French peasant, a self-taught intellectual hoisting a theatre out of ruined lives. He was profoundly non-metropolitan. He combined Brecht's truth-telling with the dream-like dissolves of cinema (*onirique *was another word I learned with him), playing games*

7

with time and space, always rooted in hard realism. He became a friend and rival of the new wave of 1960s European theatre directors – Peter Stein in Berlin, Giorgio Strehler in Milan, Yuri Lyubimov in Moscow.

Roger always wanted to write plays, and has written twenty or more, from his suicidal Ardèche history to the blues whites and reds of the Revolution, from a diptych about French seventeenth-century religious wars to Le Cochon Noir, *a play of incest, murder and despair, set during the bloody battles of the Commune. The Parisian critics were sniffy about his plays, told him to stick to directing. He was discouraged. He made elaborate films, again rubbished. He became unfashionable. A younger generation challenged his right to receive generous state subsidies when he was promoting his own work as a playwright. He strove to make his own writing poetic, and was agonised when he came to feel that, like Osborne's George Dillon, he had all the symptoms of poetry but not the disease itself. Seeking the hot-line to dream and vision, he was unquiet all his life, and still is. This feels like an obituary, but Roger's alive, living alone in Paris, writing, appearing in other people's films and plays.*

Roger reminded me of my shtetl *background. He inspired me, challenged me, lifted me out of British paths. For years after my time with him, his body language, his inflections, altered mine.*

I stayed for a year, going to rehearsals, playing bit parts and witnessing the bombs and the torture and the fascist near-takeover which marked the end of French rule in Algeria. It was a theatrical, political, European, sexual and emotional education. We went on tour to Tunisia, and wound up the tour back in Europe, in Berlin. It was 1961, the Wall was up, and at every free moment we went across to Brecht's Berliner Ensemble.

I saw Arturo Ui, *played with chilling comic force, and* Galileo, *in a set of luminous beauty. In the Berliner Ensemble canteen, a gay film-maker put his hand on my knee and asked, 'Did anyone ever tell you that you look like a Giotto?' It was time to move on. I'd stumbled by accident rather than design into two of Europe's most vital ensembles, and I was persuaded that ensemble continuity is the only way to achieve certain kinds of theatrical greatness.*

Why didn't I stay in France? Why didn't I really run away and join the circus, become a travelling player with Planchon's theatre, live in the French language? I was already halfway to integrating: I had adapted my name, which in France became Cousteau, like the deep-sea diver Jacques Cousteau. Some English friends found the name irresistibly funny, saying 'Bonjour, Monsieur Cousteau' or 'Michel Cousteau, where'd you leave your flippers, then?'

I believed, and still do, that the greatest self-discovery comes from displacement, from re-reading yourself in another language. Theatre is one of those languages, and for me then theatre spoke with a French accent. I could have gone the whole hog, I could have seized the moment, joined the ensemble, gone over to the foreigners. I didn't do it; I came back to England and began a wayward career full of detours in and out of the theatre and across the arts, into television when it was good at the start of Channel 4 and out of it when it got tidied up.

'What are you? What do you do?' people asked me. I'm a producer, I said, a commissioning editor. What I would have liked to have said is, I'm an animateur. *Lovely French word I learned. An animator: one who breathes spirit,* anima, *breath, into things. But I didn't use that word. It would have been too easy a target for that scathing British put-down sneer, 'pretentious'. So I didn't say* animateur, *and I didn't run away to France. I hadn't quite managed to join the circus. I claimed to myself and others that love of the English language, Shakespeare's stage and language, kept me from doing so.*

Scene 7: Career

I made a career. Instead of making poems and having children, I made a career. I told myself that I didn't want to repeat the same mistakes as my parents, and told others that my true children were the creative people I brought on and nurtured. Sort of true. At the Royal Shakespeare Company, which I joined a year after Peter Hall started it, I met Peter

Brook. He gave me a book about his spiritual mentor Georges Gurdjieff as a first-night present for US, *the collectively-made show we did about the Vietnam War in 1966. A book about spirit as we were doing a show about carnage and conflagration.*

I learned a lot from Brook. One big lesson was how to be quiet and give way to others in the collaborative process of making theatre. US *began with nothing. No script, just a mountain of research materials – books, papers, photos, videos – and a succession of American soldiers, avant-gardists and Christian pacifists and diplomats, British journalists, Vietnamese Buddhist monks, American draft dodgers, international peace activists, whom we questioned and taped about their Vietnam. We improvised on this material and prayed that scenes, a shape, a theme, a progression would emerge. Peter encouraged us all to leap in with ideas, and I did so, like everyone else.*

Well, not quite like everyone else. One day, Peter took me aside, and said, 'Michael, your contributions are invaluable. You are very quick and fluent. But it's precisely your speed and fluency that prevent other people having a say. Take a breath before you jump in.'

This was a shock that stopped me in my tracks. But isn't that what shocks are for? It all depends what you do with your state of being in shock. You can use a shock to begin to search for new tracks, or for no tracks at all.

Scene 8: The National Theatre

Peter Hall head-hunted me and I joined the National Theatre and we eventually opened Denys Lasdun's three theatres on the South Bank, after endless delays by builders and contractors who for months blamed each other. To mark the moment, I got my artist friend Tom Phillips invited by the National to make a poster. THE NATIONAL THEATRE IS YOURS, it read. And it could have been. I wanted the site next door to be turned over for social housing, so that not just the rich or company

It reminds me of a late poem by Brecht written in East Germany at the end of his life, when he began to know just how many millions of Communists had been betrayed and battered and murdered, when he knew that Utopias which are realised are usually Utopias betrayed, and no longer held any illusions about a radiant future. My path was a long way short of Brecht's enforced exile – 'changing countries more often than shoes'. My uprooting, my job satisfaction, the cosmopolitan I was discovering, came not from fleeing Hitler, but from the inherited reverberations of Jewish displacement.

I love this little poem because it has seen the worst of the past, is sceptical about the future, and refuses to give up.

Changing the Wheel

I sit by the roadside.
The driver is changing the wheel,
I do not like the place I have left.
I do not like the place I am going to.
So why
Do I watch him changing the wheel
With impatience?

(Translated by John Willett)

Chapter One:
A JOURNEY AND A RETURN

In July 2006 I cried out loud three times.
  Once in private, twice in public.
  Then I went to India.
  When I got back, I found I had cancer.

Friday, July 7, 2006

I'm coming home on a number 168 bus from Brixton when I wake up
to the fact that I'm in Tavistock Square, and that it's one year to the
day that a number 30 bus was blown up here. I get out and walk into
the square, past the Gandhi statue, under the tall trees making a leaf-
green canopy at dusk. A few solitary figures amble down paths or
gaze unhappily from park benches. There are a lot of television crews
about, doing dry runs for the six o'clock slot, behind them a multi-
coloured wall of flowers and tributes to the July the seventh dead.

Here's another crew, with microphones and headphones but no
camera. It's the BBC World Service, making a live radio programme
about London on this bombing anniversary, to be broadcast across
continents. A man with a baseball cap and a clipboard, he must be
the producer, approaches, recognises me, we met swimming at the
ponds on Hampstead Heath. 'Do you want to be in the programme?'
he asks. I say yes.

The interviewer is a young Muslim woman, wearing a stylish
headscarf – Hermès at a guess – and with kohl-rimmed eyes. I wait

with the two other interviewees, much younger than me, for the stopwatch to count us down to six o'clock. People in the distance are gravely inspecting the wreaths and their dedications. The trees tower over us all. Thoughts are racing through my head about what I might say, but when Ms Kohl Eyes asks me, 'What made you come into Tavistock Square?' I can't speak a word.

Unable to utter a sentence. I realise I'm crying, there's a lump in my throat, I can only get out strangled sounds. It's the sheer bloody peaceable muted Englishness of the whole scene. The tall trees. Dusk coming on. Londoners in slow motion bending over banks of flowers. I keep trying to put a sentence together, just one would be an achievement. Listeners in Cairo and Mumbai and Ramallah are being regaled with a blubbering Londoner.

Four years ago, I had a narrow escape from a suicide bomb myself.

January 2003

Netanya, Israel

I left Tel Aviv by bus an hour before the bomb went off at the Old Bus Station.

Rina, in whose house I'm staying, comes running in to say there's been an attack, and her son Itai, an orthopaedic surgeon at the trauma unit of Tel Hashomer hospital, won't be home tonight. We turn on the television, watch the handheld live footage from the poor streets around the bus station. There's a jumble of voices: they speak of two suicide bombers, they speak of a second dynamite-loaded killer waiting to catch the people running from the first explosion. A body on a pavement already shrouded, waiting for an ambulance. Bodies transported on doors, on supermarket trolleys. Commentator: 'This is the first bomb inside Israel proper since November 21.'

Whirling lights, people running, people with surgical white gloves, the camera edging close to the victims, cut away by the TV control room so they don't show the face or the wounds. A man interviewed: 'And then I saw a head rolling –'

'Spare us the plastic details,' interrupts the interviewer. Body counts rising by the minute. 'It's a neighbourhood of illegal foreign guest workers,' says Danny, my host. 'Hardly any Israeli lives in those streets. And those injury figures are probably too low. Illegal immigrants would rather run away than have their wounds treated and be deported because they have no permit.'

An hour into the live TV coverage, Islamic Jihad claims responsibility, with a reminder that fifty Palestinians have been killed by Israel in the past month, without the live coverage. The bodies keep rolling past the camera into ambulances. They're stripped to the waist, or naked to their underpants. Drip bottles of blood plasma are held over them. Cacher me'oud, *the chorus of TV journalists keeps saying: very serious.*

At breakfast time next day, Itai turns up after his night treating the wounded. Wiped out, he sits on the porch in the morning sunlight. 'There weren't just nails in the bombs, there were screws. Much harder to get out,' he says. 'Everyone I treated was a foreign worker, mostly from Thailand. Some were so badly injured they won't work again. What will happen to them? They have no money to buy a ticket back home, they send their money back to their families each month, and don't save. The private outfits that bring them over and pay them minimal wages and social security won't look after them. They'll sink to the bottom.'

In Tavistock Square, I'm still blubbing. The interviewer is loath to interrupt me; grief has its prerogatives. I struggle to draw something up from this well of wordlessness. I manage to get out a strangled phrase about this attack bringing us all closer, about looking with unaccustomed intensity at the faces of the happy kids and bent old people in the bus from Brixton. Ken Livingstone, London's mayor, may have a loose tongue, but he struck a Periclean note in his elegy for the city dead. The bombers, he is quoted as saying, saw Londoners of every race and creed come out in common grief, solidarity and humanity. We have the privilege, in this respect, to live in the greatest city on earth.

This isn't Tony Blair turning out pieties after Princess Diana's death, it's the pain of a multi-racial city, its stories cruelly ripped open like so many sardine tins. Shakespeare comes to mind; he always does. 'Man is no more but such a poor, bare, forked animal as thou art,' says Lear in the storm, and I think of the corpses of victims and rescuers, of the burned woman in the face-mask; made of paper, it could have been worn by the Trojan women in Euripides' war tragedy. And these lines from the final speech of *King Lear* seem to absorb all the cemetery sadness of this London square:

> The weight of this sad time we must obey,
> Speak what we feel, not what we ought to say.

And then I think that these elegiac sentiments are insufficient. The deaths weren't an accident, they were the result of our decisions to kill strangers and theirs to sacrifice their lives. The bombers aren't driven by 'motiveless malignity', as an eminent critic labelled the most mysterious killer in Shakespearean tragedy. They are not an army of Iagos.

Recovering my voice, I manage to say something like that, and say that the war in Iraq (and in Palestine and Afghanistan) fuelled the touchpaper of grievance and rage felt by many Muslims in Britain and around the world, holding their resentment in common with the British families whose sons have been killed and ambushed in these places far away from Tavistock Square.

The broadcast over, I make my way out of the square, nagged by questions about violence and evil, the same questions that won't let me rest when I remember Palestine, its guerrilla fighters and *shahids*. Violence is normally a last resort; but when your country, your very movements, are governed by a relentless occupier, it may become the only resort, even if unlikely to succeed because the balance of force is so weighted in Israel's favour.

Still the questions nag. If you are a young man driven by frustration and desperation, if you choose to resist, to hit back with home-made bombs, how many Israelis do you have to kill before killing becomes routine, a job like any other? Come to that, if you're a young Israeli soldier firing wire-guided missiles from your helicopter gunship, how long does it take before you treat the lives of others as disposable, nothing more than collateral damage?

Even Shakespeare could only dimly foresee the cyclical violence that disfigures our world. 'It will come / Humanity must perforce prey on itself / Like monsters of the deep,' says Albany, forced to watch his wife betray her father. Macbeth groans out the weariness of the long-distance killer caught in deadly repetition: 'I am in blood / Steeped in so far that should I wade no more / Returning were as tedious as go o'er.'

Groups of policemen pass by wearing bullet-proof jackets. It's a measure of our dwindling resistance to the drift of things that we are no longer even mildly surprised by such a sight.

Saturday, July 8, 2006

Islamexpo, a festival of all things Muslim, from the Koran to kids' stories to handicrafts to debates on 'the representation of Muslims in the media', comes to Alexandra Palace, up the hill from where I live. As I mount the steps to this Victorian edifice, coachloads of Muslim families are arriving, the car parks are filling up for this exhibition and celebration, magnanimously sponsored, 'the largest Islamic cultural event in Europe'.

The first exhibit I encounter in the vast hall is a table-top model of Israel's 'security fence,' snaking round a Palestinian town like a noose around its neck. Next to it is a model of an Israeli checkpoint, its drearily familiar features – roadblock barrier, razor-wire fences, jeeps with guns trained on travellers – miniaturised to the scale of a boy's train set. Everyone is fascinated by scale models, but I'm transfixed by this one, which gives me a God's-eye view of the reality of the Occupation.

I don't like slogans, but when I look at the wall the roadblock the future demarcation plans, the phrase 'colonial-settler state' does slip all too neatly onto the tongue.

A young man arrives next to me. We contemplate the models together. He's in his late twenties, wears a sweat-shirt and a baseball cap and is very angry. 'Animals!' he says. 'The Israelis are animals! Look how they treat us! Animals!'

I look at him, at his wife and two children. 'Are you sure they're all animals?' I say.

He won't be put off, though. 'They're all animals. If I met one now, I'd kill him for what they've done to us.'

'You would? You'd really pick up a machine-gun and –'

'Well, maybe not, but I'd do something terrible to him, with my bare hands.'

I decide to put my cards on the table.

'Look, I'm Jewish, a British Jew. I'm against the Occupation, I hate what the Israelis are doing to your people. But I don't write them all off as animals. That would be like condemning all Americans for the crimes of their army.'

The man looks at me, uncomfortable and defiant.

I move off, collect Islamic freebies, drop in on a family show by the Khayaal Theatre Company, who specialise in 'wisdom-oriented entertainment'. In what looks like a solemn gaming arcade, I take in 'the five pillars of Islam' – faith, prayer, fasting, almsgiving and pilgrimage – and on a plasma screen watch a video of crowds wheeling round the shrine at Mecca.

A young woman smiles at me from the 'Muslim Hands' stand. Behind her is another flat screen showing Palestinian walls punched with holes by Israeli shells, a bulldozer heaping up rubble that must once have been somebody's house. I think of Brecht the exile in 1940:

> This, then, is all. It's not enough, I know.
> At least I'm still alive, as you may see.
> I'm like the man who took a brick to show
> How beautiful his house used once to be.
>
> *(Translated by John Willett)*

Al Jazeera has a spacious stand. A man from their marketing department gives me a T-shirt embossed with their logo, and postcards of their martyrs: Rashi Hamid Wali (1966–2004), cameraman, killed in Iraq; Taysir Alloumi, a Spanish citizen, correspondent in Afghanistan, imprisoned by the Spanish government for 'an association with al-Qaeda'; Tarke Ayoub (1968–2003), killed when a missile – American perhaps? – slammed into the Al Jazeera offices in Baghdad; Sami al Haj, a Sudanese citizen, detained in Guantanamo since 2001.

Arabesques and geometric mazes decorate every window, wall and entrance of Ally Pally. Rounding a corner, I come upon 'Islamic Computer Games'. 'You have to know your Koran before you can play,' says a thin young man with a wispy beard. Around another corner of this labyrinthine soukh, a steward bars my way: 'You cannot come this way. It is a prayer area.'

Wednesday, July 12, 2006

The phone rings at 6.30am. It's my brother Lionel, calling from the resuscitation room of the Royal Free Hospital, where my mother – Sarah but always called Sadie – is struggling to breathe.

She'd woken with a ribbon of blood coming from the corner of her mouth, and he had rushed her to hospital. I get there just in time. A few minutes before 8am she stops breathing; the nurse turns off the oxygen cylinder. I'd got used to seeing her frowning, bewildered, frightened. Now she's calm, I stroke her smooth, cooling forehead.

The day my mother dies is also the day when I am to be presented with an honorary doctorate by London University. I don't want to pull out of this degree ceremony; going through with it will be a sign of life. My brother offers to take on the immediate tasks: the death certificate, the Jewish Burial Society, the mortuary, moving her body to the Jewish cemetery at Bushey, where she will be buried in a plot next to my father.

On the train from Waterloo to Royal Holloway College, London University's outpost at Egham, which has awarded me the degree, I realise from the newspapers that this day of my mother's death is also the day when Israel has begun the assault on Lebanon, after two of its soldiers have been captured by Hizbollah.

I look out of the window at the ravishing Thames at Staines, at Twickenham with its chorus of rugby roars stop-framed in time past. Arriving at the college in the bright sunshine, I see fluttering bunting, gleaming marquees and flocks of undergraduates looking beautiful in their gowns and mortar-boards, especially the young women. Lines of a poem by Walter de la Mare which my partner Jane recites are beating in my head:

> Look thy last at all things lovely
> Every hour. Let no night
> Seal thy sense in deathly slumber
> Till to delight
> Thou hast paid thy utmost blessing.

In the boardroom, where I am deposited, four scarlet-coated bandsmen are resting themselves and their trumpets before playing the next fanfare. Professor Dan Rebellato, the 'orator' who will trumpet my praises on the podium, arrives. I tell him about my mother's death, he puts a hand on my back.

Jane, her brother Tim, a genuine professor – of neuropsychology – and Eleni, my feisty Greek friend, arrive. I put on my billowing red gown, or frock as I prefer to think of it, tilt my medieval beret at a rakish angle, and take place in the procession through the Picture Gallery into the Chapel. 'Très camp,' I mutter to Dan, 'and très Victorian pomp.' All William Morris fleur-de-lis wallpaper and pre-Raphaelite stained glass.

We sit in the front row of the serried ranks of parents, bursting with pride as their offspring trot past. The student populace is very white, and the girls outnumber the boys by five to one. 'Always like that in drama departments,' murmurs Dan.

Finally I ascend behind him, and stand in front of the Vice-Chancellor and the Mayor of Runnymede as Dan delivers his encomium. As the list of what I've done in and out of the theatre reels out, I don't know where to look. This is turning into a day of tears and celebration mixed. I think, 'My mother would *kvell* if she was here.' To *kvell* means to swell with pride and pleasure. If your cup runneth over, you must be *kvelling*.

It's time for me to respond to Dan's speech. I've not written anything. I feel so full of things I can make a speech impromptu.

I talk about the theatre department, about the seductive beauty of English summer's days, and then change key.

'T S Eliot was wrong when he called April the cruellest month. He'd overlooked July. One year ago this month, the bombers hit London. For the past two weeks Gaza has been pulverised by Israel artillery. And yesterday in Mumbai, nameless enemies blew up a train, and the death toll to date is 200 people. Any theatre that takes no account of this, that does not show what Shakespeare called "the very age, his form and pressure" is not worth bothering about,' I say.

'And remember Hamlet said to the players that it was their job "to hold, as 'twere the mirror up to nature." The most important words in that sentence are "as 'twere". Theatre is like a mirror but it's something other than a mirror. It doesn't simply record and reflect, the way a documentary film does; it can be comic, satirical, grotesque, burlesque, fantastic. But it must somehow tap into that "form and pressure".

'Let me tell you about one such theatre,' I continue, and I tell them the story of the Freedom Theatre of Jenin.

'A young Jewish woman came from Germany to Palestine in the 1930s, married a Palestinian and started a theatre and youth arts centre in Jenin. After her death from cancer, her son Juliano took over, and is using theatre, music and art to lift the trauma the children and adolescents of Jenin undergo. In 2002, the theatre, like much of Jenin, was destroyed by the Israeli incursion, and now some of us are trying to help restart it. This theatre matters, because it teaches young men to perform in plays, not to blow themselves and Israelis up – though several of Juliano's best kids have "defected" to the armed struggle. This theatre matters, because, with all the cards stacked against it, it's trying to find something more worthwhile to do than killing. We've had enough killing, and –'

But I can't get to the end of what I want to say. I'm sobbing, I'm choking on sobs, Sadie's death has me by the throat, and I stumble to a conclusion with hundreds of eyes and close-circuit camera lenses focused on me.

Back in the boardroom, I knock back several glasses of champagne. I am now a DLitt. Tomorrow is the funeral; and then the *shiva*, the wake and the prayers for the dead, begin.

Thursday, July 13, 2006

I've cancelled the party I was going to hold in the garden to celebrate my indoctoration. I take a bus to my mum's (can't stop calling it that), getting off at Golders Green Road, which was, if I can so put it, the Mecca for shopping when I was young, and is now homogenised by chain stores and identical coffee shops, their style copied from the Tel Aviv marina. A few glimpses of the old Jewish street poke through the glittering fascias: a kosher butcher, a kosher delicatessen, a couple of bookshops selling Hebrew prayer-books and ritual objects.

Jane, who looks on these observances with the detachment of a non-Jew (indeed, a non-Christian) and a materialist, comes to my mother's house and we drive out to the cemetery, losing our way, then finding it. In a Spartan 1950s chapel, cousins and uncles and friends assemble. My sister Ruth flies in from New York. Mendel, the diminutive rabbi and father of eleven, my mother's neighbour, arrives. He used to send Sadie groups of his shy children round on Fridays bearing chicken soup and *challah*.

The funeral service begins. Lionel and I recite the Mourner's Kaddish, whose words are printed into my mind's ears from hearing them repeated a thousand times in *shul*, and yet I stumble over the syllables, the letters fluctuate, sometimes the structure of a word is clear, sometimes opaque, it will get better, by dint of repetition, over the next few days.

We walk behind the coffin to the grave, past gravestones of all shapes and sizes and prominence, denoting the wealth or status of the buried. The pale wooden coffin is lowered; the men, beginning with me as the elder son, dig clods of earth and tip them into the grave. My sister seizes the spade from my brother when he's done. The earth looks undernourished. Sadie lies next to her Mark.

Golders Green, my first universe. A date was incised into the concrete garden step: May 15 1945. Before we moved into this semi-detached in Cranbourne Gardens, at the confluence of three roads, facing a large Unitarian church and with a scatter of Jewish neighbours, I had grown up ten minutes' walk away, in another quiet Golders Green street, where my mother had lived with her mother and sister. Bella, my grandmother, was a milliner; a room downstairs was given over to feathers, trimmings and artificial flowers. There's a photograph of me aged three, in 1942, sitting in the garden by a bed of cabbages and potatoes. 'Digging for Victory,' my father wrote on the back. At the foot of the garden there was an Anderson shelter where we crouched during air raids and I claimed to identify friendly from enemy flights by the sounds of their engines.

One day a V2 rocket sailed overhead. We waited for its engine to shut down; the silence was terrifying. It dropped in a nearby street, smashing a house and killing three people. I began to have a nightmare, which lasted into my twenties, of being chased by the Gestapo through the dark streets of a World War Two town, or by plainclothes men in bulky overcoats along the labyrinthine trenches of World War One. Early on, I learned the landscapes of war.

One day in 1945 I stood with my mother in the street as hundreds of bomber planes flew overhead on their way to Germany. 'Your uncle's in one of those,' said my mum. Uncle Bernard, the first in our tribe to have further education, at Guy's Hospital, was in the medical corps, and one of the first British troops to enter the concentration camp at Belsen. He must have been devastated. Later, I heard the army had given Jewish soldiers the option whether to go to Belsen or not.

The war ended. We stayed in north London, half an hour's walk from the synagogue on High Holy Days. My father travelled daily across London to open up the shop in Tower Bridge Road, Bermondsey, where he was born and grew up, to sell clothes to mums and dads and their children. Between Golders Green and Bermondsey, the first of a series of polarities was established:

Golders Green: Jewish, home, school, shul, *library, suburbia, the Heath. Bermondsey: non-Jewish, work, the outer world, dockers, the Thames, factory workers, English working-class men and women.*

Where I grew up, a similar polarity prevailed. Across the road from the stop where I waited for the trolleybus to take me to school was a big pub, 'The Royal Oak'. None of my family ventured in, nor, as far as I knew, did any Jews. Drinking was a pagan pursuit. Cossacks did it. Pogroms ensued.

The other road from my house led to shul, *and I would walk it with my father and brother on Jewish festivals. Past the park and the rows of trim homes with their* mezuzahs *on the doorpost, past Frohwein the butcher and Susser the wine merchant, where you could buy sickly sweet ceremonial wine imported from Mount Carmel and named after it, up through streets with privet hedges to the synagogue, a 1920s would-be neoclassical temple in a street named after the ninth-century Archbishop of Canterbury, Dunstan Road.*

The pub and the shul *were the axes of the topography of my childhood and youth. Soon I added other co-ordinates. The children's library in Golders Green Road, where I learned conjuring tricks from books illustrated with engravings of venerable magicians and prestidigitators sporting Victorian moustaches and dressed in tails, which were useful for concealing bouquets of flowers made of feathers which would seemingly sprout from nowhere. The big discovery of Soho in the 'fifties, with its Indians and Jamaicans I'd never seen in Golders Green, its coffee shops (where I heard an eccentrically dressed bohemian describe his shabby top hat as 'a piss-pot hat'), its air of raffishness, rangy women and street corners, bells marked LULU or MARLENE at sidestreet front doors, and secondhand books gathering dust in the bookshops of Charing Cross Road.*

My mosaic of London began to fill out. I stood on the pavement outside my dad's shop on Saturdays – the shop made greater claims than the shul; *he had to open on Saturdays and could never keep* Shabbos *– pulling in customers with my roll-up roll-up routine. The pavement was lined with stalls, selling vegetables and household goods, lit in winter by paraffin lamps. The costermongers' cries drowned out my reedy teenage exhortations to take advantage of unrepeatable bargains. A short walk at my lunchbreak took me to Tower Bridge, its crenellated towers surmounting the busy Pool of London, then an active port. I would stand with my legs astride the break in the bridge, where it would hinge open to let tall ships through to unload goods and immigrants into the East End. Beneath my feet, the two bascules of the bridge rattled and bucked as lorries drove across. I imagined the bascules rising and the opening bridge splitting me* *in two, one half* My, *the other half* Call, *calling to each other across a chorus of ships' horns.*

My father had grown up in Bermondsey, in rooms above the shop where he was now, as the fascia proclaimed, a 'children's outfitter'. I never understood why his parents had settled in Southwark and not across the bridge in Whitechapel or Stepney, where most Jews arriving from Russia and Eastern Europe lived. Maybe the rents were cheaper. As it was, my dad was doubly separated: from the middle-class Jews aspiring to Englishness by wearing bowlers and top hats in Golders Green synagogue, and from the seethe of Yiddish-speaking working-class Jews of the East End, the heartbeat of Eastern Europe in Stepney and Limehouse. He was an outsider to both communities, a stranger to each congregation.

In Harold Pinter's *The Homecoming*, the play of his which most haunts me, the mother (named just once: Jessie) is airbrushed from the play. Dead when the action begins, she's only reincarnated in her husband Max's recollections, for the most part safely idealised, but at one point lurching into violent dislike.

> Mind you, she wasn't such a bad woman. Even though it made me sick just to look at her rotten stinking face. I gave her the best bleeding years of my life, anyway.

Max looms large, he seizes the foreground, he blocks her out. Maybe that's why I am so stirred by this play; for me, Max's ambivalence, his idealisation and his loathing, are part of the ultimate 'family romance' – Freud's description of one of the primal mechanisms of families, the child's need to wrench himself from the family, see women in a sexual light, and become not just a son, but a man. *The Homecoming* seemed a perfect fit – allowing, of course, for Pinter's wild comic enlargements. Pinter's characters don't button down their emotions as the sufferers in Terence Rattigan's dramas do. They allow their passions and hostilities to come shooting out, often with the ferocity of projectile vomit.

SADIE

My mother giggling, then sad. Her mother Bella, sad at the end of her days. Bella saying, whispered, 'I remember tomorrow as if it was yesterday.' Or was it 'I remember yesterday as if it was tomorrow'? Either way, the mind hanging loose, hovering across her face, her weary body. The face of the deep. And darkness moved across the face of the deep, as my mother Sadie and her sister Maisie sat by her bed and Grandma Bella briefly became an oracle, after a lifetime as a milliner, making felt hats trimmed with fake flowers and fruit.

My mother giggling. 'Laughing eyes, they used to call me at school,' she'd say. Another way of eroding her. Her laughter was shouldered out by the end, after ten dutiful years looking after my father, Mark, as he sunk into senile dementia. My mother shy; my father, aggressive, with waiters, hotel receptionists, servants, salespeople – of which he was one, though of a superior caste, he thought. His bossy behaviour in unfamiliar environments said, 'Look, I'm not just an employee, I'm in retail, I'm a businessman, I have my own shop. Treat me with respect.'

My mother giggling, in a ballgown. In the 'thirties, Sadie and Mark went to tea dances. It was the age of Ambrose and his Orchestra, of Victor Silvester and Fred Astaire, my father's hair brilliantined like Fred's, his gliding steps aiming to emulate Fred.

My mother giggling in the kitchen.

Why can't I get my father out of Sarah's story?

My mother, giggling in the kitchen. Her territory. She made a cacophony of cooking pots as she worked, as if to assert her presence there. She had relinquished her place in the larger world when her father died just as she was due to go to university. She had to give up her place; it was the 1930s, and her family needed another breadwinner. She could have been an avid undergraduate, spreading her wings in worlds beyond suburban Golders Green. But there are so many could-have-beens for Jewish mothers of her generation.

She mourned her father all her life. He died of cancer not yet fifty. He'd been a bespoke tailor in Soho, one of the elite of the profession, a dab hand

29

at double-breasted suits, pleated waistbands and luminous linings. Sadie loved his dapper image. When my father came along, seemingly forceful, though racked inside with his own family rages and guilts – but I want to keep him out of this, my mother's territory – she succumbed. His combativity strengthened her; her softness gentled him.

'You're making love with the man next door!' he screamed in his later dementia, a seventy-year-old man with a crazy brain. 'I'll catch you at it, you slut!' The Mark she had married was disappearing into his paranoid disease. Once he ran out into the street in search of her in the act of cuckolding him, kicked over milk bottles and had to be rescued by the rabbi who lived on the other side.

I want him out of the picture.

She went to adult education literature classes when I was at Oxford. She wanted to discuss an essay she'd written about D H Lawrence. But I was going through my own Laurentian torment, trying to fall in love with a girl without feeling I was betraying my mother; a discussion about Sons and Lovers *was the last thing I needed.*

Sarah made chopped liver – Jewish ambrosia; her chicken soup was a golden essence of poultry distilled, Olympian nectar from a Jewish mother. My father had formulaic compliments for my mother's cooking each Friday night around the Shabbos *candles: 'Sadie, your soup tastes like wine, your meat like butter' – though associating butter with meat would have offended the dietary laws, of course. She also had the gift of darker flavours: her* borscht *was a deep purple ambiguous liquid that played sweet–sour games with your taste buds.*

My occluded mother. Why are these tastes so much more vivid than her own sweet-sad face? Are recipes her most lasting legacy?

When my mother went to shul, *to the synagogue in Golders Green, she'd arrive after my father and brother and I had already been in the all-male congregation downstairs for an hour,* dovening: *praying in a minor-key chant with a self-hypnotic rocking back and forth. Sadie would appear upstairs among all the women, wearing a rakishly-tilted hat her milliner mother would have made at her best. Looking up at her, surrounded by other elegantly-dressed, perfumed women, I could imagine a family romance with her myself.*

When I won a scholarship to Oxford, my father wanted me to read law, so I could have a 'profession' like the other bright Jewish boys, who were knocking themselves out to become solicitors, doctors or accountants. 'But I want to read English literature,' I said, inflamed by my reading of Dylan Thomas and John Donne and T S Eliot. 'You can always study English later,' he said. I knew it was a trap. I'd never get off the treadmill if I studied law. My mother could see that too; though she was not too hot at standing up for herself, she took a stand for her son, and backed me.

In her last months, I went to sit with her at weekends, in her nineties, unable to walk, tilting into all-day sleep in her chair, her memory reaching out to words and phrases that were always beyond reach.

I staged Peter Handke's threnody on the insanity and eventual suicide of his mother, A Sorrow Beyond Dreams, *at the National Theatre. Gawn Grainger, an actor of fierce emotion and economy, captured Handke's desperate search for meaning in his mother's diminished life. Handke allows glints of poetry, sharp remembered details to peep through: 'from her childhood days my mother had a swollen scar on her index finger; I held onto it when I walked beside her.'*

Sadie slept, jaw slack, dreaming, waking up in panic, subsiding again into sleep. Like candles, her brain-cells were blowing out one by one. When she goes, I thought, will I be Jew enough to remember to kindle yahrzeit *– memorial – candles for her?*

MARK

When my father reached his fifties, he sold his children's outfitter's shop in Bermondsey, to open a dry-cleaning shop nearer home. I meant to buy and keep the fascia sporting my grandfather's name above the shopfront. The letters were bevelled and gold-leafed, seemingly chiselled out of a long, shiny black slab. It was monumental. On the rare occasions I drove past 108 Tower Bridge Road, I vowed to stop, go in, introduce myself as the son of the previous owner, and do a deal with the new one for the fascia.

I never did; one day I went past and saw the new proprietor's name displayed, in much inferior lettering. My grandfather's name must have wound up in some dump, the long slab shattered.

This made me think about Kristallnacht *in Germany in 1938, when Jewish shops and shopkeepers were smashed up. The shopkeepers, for whom an imposing frontage on a German high street would have been evidence of accession to the German family, were terrified. Now I couldn't even take steps to preserve my grandfather's name-plate, though I wondered, what I would have done with that mammoth A. KUSTOW & SONS sign. Where would I have put it? It would have needed a big garage to itself, a boathouse, a long loft. Still, I regretted its disappearance. It had served my family like a heraldic banner, and now there was little left to connect me with my father's father.*

Among the many fears which underlay his aggressiveness, Mark had bad memories of the goyische *men of Bermondsey, especially the dockers, big blokes strong enough to lift heavy cargo from the ships tied up at the wharves of the Pool of London. He remembered the dock so crammed with ships that you could cross the Thames by walking from one deck to another. He saw men shoving and crowding each morning to get a job from the foreman, and heard about bribes and threats to ensure that the strongest got their way. The story that seared him, though, happened in the General Strike of 1926, when dockers came out in solidarity with the striking miners. Pitched street battles between strikers and police broke out in Bermondsey, with the brawny dockers leading the attacks. My father, who was eighteen at the time, remembered a huge docker coming into the pub on the corner, downing a pint and smashing the pint-glass on the counter. 'He took the glass and rushed out,' my father told me. 'Soon I saw him in the midst of the battle. He crept up to a mounted policeman and suddenly screwed the glass into the horse's flank. It whinnied in pain, reared and the policeman was thrown to the ground and trampled on.'*

When he retired and his mind started to fragment, Mark sat at the glass-topped dining table and began to turn out drawings and water-colours, of vases of flowers and landscapes. Not much of his bold, shop-

window-shaping self in them; he fell back on a fine-tipped mapping pen and black ink to make outlines, which he then filled in with watercolour. It reminded me of painting by numbers, which was apt, since in many ways my father had grown up living by numbers and constraints. He needed to carve out worlds with a definite outline; the fluidity of watercolour or the slow pace of oil painting were not for him. He might have been good at chiselling gold letters into shopfronts.

When I think of my father and his parents, I see him locked in furious struggles, especially with his mother; she had him by the balls. It's a familiar immigrant story. His mother Annie and father Alexander, Russian-Jewish émigrés, had met in London, in some transitory refugee location. They'd made a hasty marriage of convenience, which she soon regretted. 'She came from a better class of family than his,' whispered malicious family gossips. 'She'd never have looked twice at him back home.'

My father had a deep well of depression, which he tried to keep at bay by being bossy and busy and throwing temper fits. This wore him out, and he succumbed to senile dementia, slowing down to a silent standstill, taking for ever for the simplest tasks. Finding it hard to bear his shrinkage, I wrote to him on Christmas Eve 1990:

> *Dear Dad,*
>
> *There must be a thousand things you want to say and do, and your mind and body won't let you. When you tell me how long it takes you to get dressed, you're telling me how frustrated you are. When I look at your eyes staring into the distance, I can only imagine what you're thinking. For a man like you, who's been in charge of his own territory all his life, to feel helpless now must be hard to take.*
>
> *Dad, what I want to say isn't about the present so much as the past. I want to tell you that, however much you may recriminate with yourself for doing things wrong, you've certainly given me many more positive than negative things. The image and example of a fighter, to start with. A feeling for old London – Bermondsey and old brick walls and the river – and through that, an interest in history.*

A love of stalls and street markets. Drive, push, zest, showbiz. How to handle a paintbrush. The pleasure of selling things: I like saying to my peers that I'm the son of a shopkeeper.

I'm even grateful – now, anyway – for the struggles I had with you to find my own way, against your ideas of the path I should follow. A friend told me he thinks his son lacks vim and vigour because the son's career has already been hugely achieved by his successful father. I chose a different field from you – theatre, culture, the arts, words – perhaps in rebellion against you, and that rebellion gave me energy. In different ways, my brother and sister also benefited: the struggle gave us dynamism as well as neurosis. You should finally stop blaming yourself for what you imagine you've done to your children. We are what we make of what we get – genetically, psychologically, economically, and culturally.

At Oxford I sometimes fantasised about belonging to a genteel, well-behaved, cultivated English family. That was a wet dream, and I'm not sorry to have grown up in an unruly, non-English one.

There are, of course, many things I regret – a lot of them, I now see, due to the war and being a war baby and you having all the strains and stresses of keeping the show on the road during the blitz. But I'm sorry we never went to a football match together, that I couldn't see you as part of a group of men friends in a pub, a club, or whatever. Going to shul *together was always good, though, and I think you felt good with us, even surrounded by those self-important Jews in bowler hats. Good too were: drawing things with you, reciting gems of Eng Lit from the battered copy of* Bell's Elocution *you bought, going to the East End with you and watching you bully late-delivering manufacturers. And don't forget how many popular songs I learned from you –* I Left My Sugar Standing In The Rain And My Sugar Melted Away, Ain't She Sweet, Mammy *and all the other Al Jolson songs you sang as you were shaving in the bathroom heavy with the smell of your shit – you couldn't start your day without dumping a massive load.*

In the *Haggadah*, the book of the Passover service, the *Seder* (which sometimes coincides with Easter, sometimes doesn't, depending on the lunar cycle), four kinds of son are described. The Intelligent One. The Wicked One. The Simple One. And the One Who Does Not Know How To Ask. The first wants to know chapter and verse on the duties demanded by God. The second wants to know what the others round the table mean by the whole religious service, and speaks as if he was an outsider, as if it didn't concern him. The third just asks 'What is all this?' His father replies with a verse from Exodus: 'By strength of hand, God brought us out of Egypt, out of the house of bondage.' And to the last, who is either too young or too over-awed to ask a question, the father adds, 'You must open yourself up', and another Exodus quote: 'And thou shalt tell thy son that day, saying, It is because of what God did for me when I came out of Egypt.'

I loved the *Seder*. It seemed to me a festival of liberation, the emancipation of the Jews from enslavement to Pharaoh in Egypt, and that had a metaphorical as well as a historical force. I made one other line in the service a personal motto: 'In every age, every Jew shall behave as if he or she had just been released from Egypt.' Cherish your freedom, in other words; relish your reclaimed life; respect the freedom of others. Maybe this qualifies me as an Intelligent Son.

My father Mark was the second eldest of four sons, and the Haggadah *might have filed him as the Simple Son, for he allowed his mother to wrap him round her little finger and did her bidding uncomplainingly. Ahead of him was Leonard, seen as the family's wheeler-dealer, who dealt in everything from industrial safety goggles to mansions on the Côte d'Azur. Probably the Wicked One. He earned quick money in dubious deals and spent it on glitzy* shikses — *a racist word meaning 'non-Jewish women,' forbidden seductive temptresses — and silk ties from Sulka in Mayfair.*

Next down from my father was Bernard, the only one to prise himself out of the reiterations of family life and family voices, by getting an education. The Intelligent One, for sure. He studied medicine at

Guy's hospital, became a GP and increasingly a private practitioner in Willesden, complaining that his largely Jewish patients were driving him crazy, taking his kishkes – entrails – out with their demands. He schmoozed them relentlessly just the same, went to their weddings and barmitzvahs, pocketed their gratefully tendered cheques.

He always seemed dissatisfied, not only with his patients but also with his children. He was especially disappointed with his son, Danny, who became lead guitarist for the Tom Robinson band in the 'seventies, married 'out' to a tiny Scottish girl, had a child and then a massive breakdown, which required hospitalisation. It didn't do much good; Danny was now a shadow of the thrilling, exuberant musician he had been. I went to see him in some kind of sanatorium in Hampshire where he had rigged up his guitar and amps in a barn. He played a bit: the gift was not dulled, though on the way to being so.

I'd always liked Danny. He was the least embourgeoisé of the family, and it occurs to me that although he was several years younger, we stood in the same position in our respective families: third-generation immigrant offspring, second-generation English.

Dissatisfaction was Uncle Bernard's default emotion. Nothing that befell him was good enough, including his gifted son.

Last in the family matrix was Felix. The Simple Son, perhaps, certainly the most straightforward of the four brothers, he had a sunny disposition and a sweet tenor singing voice. He must also have had the patience of a saint, for he worked his whole life side by side with my bossy father. They developed something of a double-act. The mums of Bermondsey used to save up to buy a tailor-made suit for their apple-of-the-eye sons, paying in instalments. My father and Felix had a time-honoured routine to welcome in mother and son for the final fitting after the last payment had been made. Mark would tug the jacket about, so that the shoulder 'sat' correctly, and the trousers rested on the hips. Then he would stand back, gaze admiringly at the embarrassed kid, turn to his mum and say, 'There you are, missus. All he needs is a bar of chocolate down the front.' The mother would cluck with laughter and, beaming, escort her teenage *wonder-boy out of the shop. She did not hear Felix turn to my father and say, 'Mark, a miracle! It fits!' To which my father would invariably bat back, with Max Wall solemnity, the politically incorrect punchline, 'He must be a cripple.'*

My father's servitude to his mother, and his struggles against it began when his father started to go absent from the shop, drinking and running after women. With Leonard gallivanting round the West End (which I envisaged an El Dorado of neon signs, fairy lights and spangled women) and with Bernard and Felix too young to help, Grandma Annie fastened on my father. He ran errands for her, shlepped *parcels and bales of cloth on chilly open-topped buses from the East End, did stocktaking, descending into the dank cellar, despatched orders in brown-paper parcels, beautifully wrapped, climbed wearily up the bare stairs to the cold bedroom. 'And she never thanked me,' he said, on countless occasions. 'I never got a smile out of her. She took me for granted. Because she was unhappy, everyone round her had to be miserable as well.'*

Friday, July 14, 2006

I am up and about early, the birds chirping in the trees that surround our garden. Unable to think or write, I potter about, filing papers, replacing books. I decide to put on some music. Jimmy Rushing, the big blues singer, backed by a Kansas City band. He lifts his voice like a crane hoisting a cargo, it rolls and rides across the striding band. I sing along with *Ain't Nobody's Business If I Do* and then he starts blues, sad, dusky, beginning with the words 'In The Evenin'...' – and that's it, the floodgates open, and I'm streaming tears here in my workplace, drowning the birdsong, something erupts, it's released, it's out. The second time this month.

Peter Brook rings from France. 'I'm calling to take your temperature,' he says. I was due to leave today for Avignon, where I would meet him and see his latest production, but I've cancelled that. I try to explain why it was Jimmy Rushing who triggered my tears, Peter tells me not to worry about not coming to Avignon, but to 'stay with what's happening, and do as little as possible'. His advice reminds me of Shakespeare's Macduff, who, being told that his wife and children have been murdered by Macbeth's thugs, breaks down into incoherent weeping. 'Dispute it like a man,' his companion says.

'I shall do so,' replies Macduff, 'but I must feel it as a man.'

I am trying to feel my mother's death as a man.

An hour later Pamela Howard, a designer and director with whom I've worked for years, and who has herself just lost her father, phones. 'You're an orphan,' she says. I'd never thought of that; being orphaned was something that happened to little children in Dickens novels. But it's a fact. As the first-born child of the Kustows, I am in the front line. Ahead, Death waits. For years, my mother and father walked ahead of me, protecting me from a direct hit. Then my father died. Only my mother stood between me and the grinning reaper. Now she's gone.

I have no more human shield.

August / September 1939

My father planted the sperm that was to become me in my mother's womb in March 1939. By the summer, as the drums of war grew more insistent, he moved her out of London to a safer place, a succession of rented rooms in villages near Newbury and Chippenham. He remained on duty in London, keeping an eye on the flat in which they had begun their married life and going every day to open his shop in Tower Bridge Road.

Other Jewish people went there too – her mother Bella, her sister Maisie, his mother Annie, and friends of theirs. A small outpost of Jewish evacuees in a picture-postcard English village called Christian Malford.

They wrote to each other feverishly. If letters had voices and I had had X-ray ears, these are the words of Sadie and Mark I would have heard from inside the womb.

Sadie darling (my chuchie), Sidney Reitman phoned and he has fixed up a room in the next house to Cissie. So I will come down by the first possible train on Sunday and take you there. At least you will be near somebody of your own class and also have quite a few Jewish friends staying nearby.

Mark, down here you get into the habit of thinking things are not real, until you hear the wireless or read the papers... Perhaps a miracle will happen and we can all be saved from this horror that hangs over us. Look after yourself, darling, and have plenty to eat, for my sake.

I lay in bed this morning thinking about all the happy times we had together from our honey moon. That night you came down in your lovely black dinner gown, you were marvellous – first and last skiing lesson, so hot it was I took my shirt off – skating on the lake, the day you had your hair dressed, the Casino, Paris, Folies Bergère, naked girls, sea sick, back home... I was so happy to be near you, to see you and hear your voice. This separation is very bad just as we were settling down and entering our lives sweetly.

Darling, when you come Sunday, please God, could you remember to bring a large, new cardboard box or a suitcase to put the baby's things in? ...bring as many of the baby's things that I shall need right away (but don't overdo it). You don't have to bring the blankets, just the napkins, nightdresses, shawl, etc. I should have everything ready by a month before, that is, two weeks' time.

I phoned Chilprufe yesterday. They still haven't got the nightdresses. Last night I went to the Trocette Cinema in Tower Bridge Road and saw for the third time Captain Blood. *I listened to a play called* Twenty Years

After, *in it a man and girl were very much in love with each other. They expressed each other's thoughts so beautifully that I felt like getting up and writing the words down to send to you my love.*

Please God I hope we shall be together very soon, to enjoy a happy life together, with our baby Please God. When we have the baby it will bring us a happiness that we have never experienced.

Is our baby behaving itself? I'm sure it's a fidget like its father.

August 30: I spent the most miserable evening of my life last night. After you phoned I went to the flat. When I went in I felt like crying... Everything here is on edge. People walk about with a heavy look and you can feel the tension in the air.

I knew you would be upset staying at the flat alone I felt it inside me all the time – and cannot bear to think of our home without you and me together in it.

Leonard joined the anti-aircraft corps yesterday and he went away this morning, he is not a full soldier, he will be stationed at Strathan and will have to carry out training for 4 weeks in a way... You know Leonard he can turn the whole army inside out, he's already made some business with the Chief Commander and bamboozled him so much that the poor fellow doesn't know whether he's in the Army or Navy

Business, of course, is very slow... I think myself there WON'T BE WAR everyone says that if he does not strike until now, he won't do so at this stage.

I wish the time would should fly for the baby to come, please God, – it is only a few weeks now, at times I have a great thrill and excitement going through me, I am longing to see him and dream of the moment, please God, when you see him for the first time and hold him in your arms.

This evening just as my father and I were driving to the East End a terrible fire broke out at the Wholesale Fitting Company in Commercial Street. It was a terrific blaze.

Mother and Maisie have just come back with the news, that if anything, the situation is more serious, as Hitler still insists on Danzig and Polish corridor and will not give in. All of a sudden my nerves gave way, angel, and I ran upstairs and lay on the bed, crying 'I want you, Mark, I can't be without you, sweetheart' – the loneliness inside you is unbearable – it hurts so much I had to cry and cry to relieve it…to be without you, even for a day, is agony, sweetheart, I need to talk to you, look at you, as much as I need to eat.

Don't forget to have a gasmask and socks, have a bath and change your underwear and socks, you will feel better if you look bright and put a face on it. The baby sends a nice big kick, just to remind you he's on the way.

I don't sleep so well lately, dear, (that of course is the baby mostly – it usually is so in the last few weeks) but when I do, I dream of you, I lie in the dark, thinking and imagining what is going to happen to us and hoping, praying with all my might that this mockery of life will soon end. Darling, don't forget when you come Friday, please God, to wear a dark suit and to bring a hat, because, this being Yom Kippur, you should not wear light clothes.

I have made up my mind. I cannot do without you for much longer, I will stick it out until the baby comes, please God, and then I am coming home to you, darling…unless life in London becomes too dangerous to be borne, which God forbid. I don't see why we should be deprived of our happiness any longer. As long as we are spared, dear, I intend to share everything with you, all the joys and sorrows which are coming to us, we are going to experience together, otherwise, to me, life itself is without meaning, merely existence without point, as is time now. Yesterday I went to the pictures, the Joan Crawford picture was quite ordinary, except for the skating scenes, which were really wonderful. P.S. Will you bring me some nice, clean tissue paper to wrap the baby's things in.

On the letter I can see the lipstick imprint she has sent him.

Chapter Two:
FAMILY STRIFE

Sunday, July 16, 2006

A death in the family takes the stopper out of the bottle; all kinds of feelings jump out. Sitting in my mother's garden with my brother Lionel, his Israeli wife Ilana and my sister Ruth, I find myself attacked for what I've written and said about Israel. What this adds up to: a handful of articles and letters to the press criticising Israel's treatment of the Arabs; a screening at the London School of Economics of a film about Palestinians from the West Bank revisiting the sites where their villages used to be; and, most offensive to my brother and sister and, it seems, to most of our relatives and their friends, a public letter in which I and a dozen other British Jews renounced our automatic 'right of return' to Israel.

This was a privilege granted in 1950 by Ben Gurion's government, whereby 'every Jew has the right to come to this country as an *oleh* (a settler)'. In 1950 this law made sense against the sombre background of the Holocaust. But by the year 2000, when we unhappy Jews signed our letter of renunciation, things had changed. The immigration of Soviet Jews had been the last sizeable emigration of Jews from exile to Zion. In what Bernard Wasserstein calls 'the vanishing diaspora', Jewish communities in America, Latin America, France, and Britain stayed put, assimilated, visited Israel as tourists and made donations to hospitals and universities, but did not settle in Zion.

So, fifty years after its conception, the Law of Return had become an act more symbolic than real. Except for the Palestinians, who had once lived in what was now Israel. They had no right of return, no matter how many years of occupancy they could prove, and no compensation.

This disparity of treatment, though logical in a Jewish state preserving its demographic dominance, had driven us to write our letter of renunciation. To my brother and sister and sister-in-law that afternoon, it seemed nothing less than an act of hubris, an incendiary provocation.

'I've never said this before, Michael,' says Lionel, 'but you should never have signed that letter. It was a slap in the face to your own people. And to the survivors of the Holocaust.'

'It might have been if we'd called for the repeal of the Law of Return,' I say. 'But we were just a bunch of Jews who said, we don't want to benefit from this law, when the people who lived there before can't do so.'

'Have you lived in Israel? Do you understand ordinary Israelis – not just artists and intellectuals?' Lionel's wife Ilana asks sharply. 'Have you any idea how much ordinary Israelis long for peace?'

'You've cut yourself off with that stupid letter,' adds Lionel. 'Do you know how many friends and business colleagues ask me, "What's he up to, that crazy brother of yours?"'

I try to reply to what is beginning to feel like a concerted attack from my relatives, and in a larger sense from my extended Jewish family. They're turning on a renegade, almost a blasphemer.

'What you're all saying adds up to "Who do you think you are?", to "What gives you the right to pass judgement, to criticise Israel?" I have just as much right as any Diaspora Jew. You know I don't want Israel "driven into the sea". I want it to survive. But being a British Jew doesn't disqualify me from being critical. And of course Hizbollah must be stopped. But unleashing a military juggernaut, blitzing a neighbouring society, providing world television with horrific images night after night will simply stack up trouble for years to come. Israel's collective punishment is setting up a catastrophe for itself. And for Jews everywhere. For the rest of us.'

But I'm getting nowhere. I've become their Cain, and they're all angry with me. Well, so it goes. 'Remember Rabbi Hillel and his two questions,' I say. 'First question: If I am not for myself, who will be for me? Second question: But if I am only for myself, what am I?'

The day winds down, shadows reach across the lawn. The *minyan*, the quorum, gathers for mourning prayers. There have to be at least ten men to make a *minyan*. We easily pass that number. Mendel, the rabbi who lives next door, arrives with two young men and a little package wrapped in cloth. They choose a small table as a makeshift altar and unwrap the package. It contains the Torah, the scrolls, hand-written on parchment, of the Old Testament, which every Jew is taught to regard as sacrosanct. Jewish history and legend tell many stories of martyrdom undergone to preserve the Book, from medieval pogroms to torture by the Inquisition, from the defiant raising aloft of the Torah in the confines of the ghetto, to its invocation in the death camps.

Now we have a Torah in our dining room. The service begins, led by Mendel, chanting the prayers no louder than a whisper, a stream of barely audible syllables with occasional phrases plucked out for emphasis, all the while rocking back and forth, flexing the knees, bowing the head. It's contagious: I find myself wanting to join in, but display independence by rocking from side to side. Like a jazz singer, it strikes me, or like Jimmy Witherspoon, or like Mick Jagger in his quieter moments.

The prayer-book I'm holding is written in words I still recall from my childhood, remember in an Ashkenaz, German and northern European, rather than a Sephardic, Spanish and southern European, accent. *Somech noflim, oo-ro-fay cholim, oo-mateer asoorim,* my favourite riff from the prayer called *Amidah* ('standing'). Its parallelisms and rhymes went straight into my cerebral cortex, as did its meaning: 'You support the falling, heal the sick, liberate the bound.' I'm feeling a bit like a falling creature myself today.

The dipping and bowing come to an end, and we three – my sister has been invited to leave the women's section of the room to join us – sit on special low chairs provided for mourners. Family and friends file past, shake hands, hug and mutter, 'Wish you a long life.' Formulaic it may be, but the value of formulae is to let people say something when words fail them.

Monday, July 17, 2006

If it weren't for my mother's death and the *shiva* I would have been in Avignon now, seeing plays in the Palais des Papes, whose vast open-air stage and young audiences shrill with excitement first lured me into theatre four decades ago.

Now the bombs are falling on Lebanon. What can a man, an individual, do in this wind-tunnel of war? I talk with Peter Brook, who is still in Avignon with his actors, and we come up with the idea of another letter about the war, an international letter, for publication in the *New York Times*, for it is America that holds the key to a cease-fire.

There now begins a ten-day chase after names, pulling in our connections, from New York to Jenin, Petersburg to Tel Aviv. I spend hours trying to get to Steven Spielberg; his name would carry weight. Tony Kushner isn't answering, nor is Glenda Jackson, nor is Daniel Barenboim, who may be in Berlin or Chicago or Seville. Peter, on his mobile phone, calls me three or four times a day, anxious as time is slipping past and the number of civilian casualties in Israel and Lebanon relentlessly rises. We keep on amending the text of the letter, which is becoming a plea and a redefinition of moderation from makers and thinkers. 'Moderation in this struggle is dismissed as weakness. But if people cannot reassert it, the attractive slogans of violence will take over. Is it too late for us to recognise that a moderate attitude is not a weak and spineless compromise, that it makes undeniably strong demands on honest feeling and pitilessly clear thought?'

I'm beginning to think I've taken on too much. As well as the *New York Times* letter, there's the aftermath of my mother's death. My sister, with characteristic energy, has flung herself into the task of putting Sadie's belongings in order. Her bustle – filling bin bags with clothes to be donated to charity; writing labels showing which objects she'd like to have – all this grates on Lionel, who feels it as hostility.

I've also agreed to put together at short notice a sequence of readings for a Trafalgar Square meeting organised by the Palestine Solidarity Campaign, *Voices For Lebanon and Palestine*. Over one week, with the help of Cass Harwood, I compile the script, clear the rights and cast the actors. Elegies for Beirut from Robert Fisk and Zena El-Khallil. Adrian Mitchell's *To Whom It May Concern*, originally written about the lies being told about the Vietnam war, but, alas, as apt for all the wars that have followed. Poems by Pinter and by a Palestinian woman in a British jail. A monologue by Terry Jones for a member of the 'Armageddonist Party', grateful that death and destruction are now assured for years to come.

I e-mail a flier for this event to a group of friends, most of them Jewish. By return I get angry replies accusing me of helping Israel's enemies.

'You are a very creative, interesting, engaging man and I like you a lot,' says the first friend, a psychotherapist. 'But when it comes to the Middle East and things Jewish, you seem to become unbalanced, almost unhinged. Are you fighting your brother? Your mother, your previous Israeli wife? Personal demons yet unspoken?'

'It says in the Torah that one must love all one's fellow Jews. I think of Jews, yourself included, and I find that hard, when I see you organising a demo that gives succour to our enemies.'

The second rebuke comes from the playwright Arnold Wesker, who I have known since I was a student. We've had a long-running argument about Israel and the Arabs, and our dialogue continues in my head as I read his words.

'I'm so sad,' he writes, 'to see you among Bin Laden's barmies, as there used to be Lenin's and Stalin's idiots, those "friends" of the Soviet Union who would visit and return with their eyes shining over.'

'Dear friend,' I answer, 'I haven't become a fellow-traveller of the Palestinians. I am and remain a British Jew who can't stand what's being done to Lebanese children.'

'How on earth can you be part of a demonstration,' he continues, 'that makes no reference to the culpability of Hezbollah and the hundreds of thousands of Israelis living in shelters while businesses flounder unattended?'

'Businesses floundering? Who's looking after the shop?' I'm tempted to say. 'Is that the worst calamity to hit the people of this wretched region? And yes, the performance in Trafalgar Square won't ignore the loudmouths of Hizbollah, including one of their leaders who referred to Jews as a tumour and a cancerous growth.'

'Oh, God!' he concludes. 'Why can't I be on the politically correct side for once in my life? I'd feel so much happier.' But I don't feel any happier and certainly less comfortable producing a performance for the Palestinians at this time – not commentating and point-scoring from the sidelines. I hope our friendship will survive this argument.

Saturday, July 22, 2006

On the stage in Trafalgar Square there are several Jews, and at least one of them, the actor Henry Goodman, an outstanding Shylock at the National Theatre, is being mug-shot by *The Jewish Chronicle*. Waiting to go on and read a poem I've written, Henry looks thoughtful. A few minutes later, he looks more than thoughtful, he looks anguished. But he goes on and hits an attentive audience with the poem which my contradictions and unease have wrung out of me:

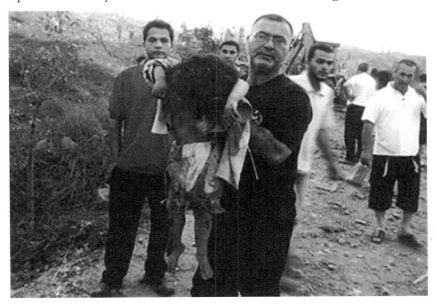

The Guernica of Lebanon

You ask: who will paint the Guernica of Lebanon?
not 'our correspondent' broadcasting live
standing in a rubbleheap
that was once a shaded boulevard
not the hand-held lens
ducking in fear from a close-up explosion

popping up again to capture
a baby's twisted body in Beirut
tossed aside like a used tissue.

Where is the Lebanese Picasso?
Stupid question: running for his life.
In his place, installation artists
build rubble-castles with their bunker-busters
debris-artists document the devastation.

The lights have gone out, the television's stopped.
Who will paint the gape-mouthed victims
screaming in the jagged light of an oil-lamp?
No-one will paint the victims.
They don't sit still for a sitting.
They have to get somewhere else.
Anywhere but Lebanon. Fast.

'We will grind the guerrillas into the ground,'
says the leader in Jerusalem.
Lacking the bulk of his predecessor
he must try harder to project power.
But why does everything he says
sound like a speak-your-weight machine?

Who am I to speak?
I am a Jew
like the John Wayne impersonator in Jerusalem
he an Israeli Jew, I a London Jew
who cannot take what is being done this summer
to Lebanese families.

It is not intended, say the emollient voices
It is collateral, say the indignant voices
It is regrettable but it must be done

that our people may be safe
in the land of milk and honey
say the voices of victimhood.

I hear you say
'Our towns our schools our hospitals our railways
are targeted by enemy missiles.
We have to cripple that enemy for good
smash his limbs like a baby's
You have a problem with that?'

Yes, I have a problem.
Neither your sophistry nor your bombardment
come from any inheritance I recognise as Jewish.
Every spray of shrapnel
nail-bomb
ball-bearing canister
'anti-personnel device' fresh from the arms fair
sucks away the marrow
from the good things Jews have given to the world
which now lie under the rubble with infant corpses.

Only one word makes sense: Stop. Stop. Stop.

The actor's reading is interrupted by an attempt to set fire to an Israeli flag right in front of the stage.

Samuel West quietens the audience by reading an extract from Daniel Barenboim's Reith Lectures about music and politics.

The genuine and original idea of the renewal of Jewish settlement in Palestine has been totally overwhelmed and diverted by forces that believe that power rules the social and political destiny of humanity. But this is a land for two people, with opposing narratives, but of necessity equal rights.

It is essential to understand the difference between strength and power. Power itself has only one kind of strength, which is that of control. In Beethoven, Brahms or Wagner, even the most powerful chord has to allow the inner voices to be heard, otherwise it has no tension, only brutal aggressive power. You must hear the opposition, the notes that oppose the main idea.

Music to me is sound with thought. Music speaks to all parts of the human being. Music teaches us that everything is connected.

And then on comes Shadia Mansour, a sombre and contained Palestinian singer, who rouses the audience to swaying, handclapping, painful affirmation.

Meanwhile, for our *New York Times* letter we now have six Nobel laureates, Barenboim (who said 'yes' immediately once our letter reached him), a former UN envoy to Iraq, film director Costa-Gavras and Nick Hytner, director of the National Theatre. I feel like a quick-change artist hopping between Trafalgar Square and *The New York Times*. Peter Brook is getting impatient, but it can't go any faster. Finally, two weeks after it started, the letter appears.

'No words are strong enough to capture what is happening in Lebanon, Gaza and Israel,' it begins,

> Yet the world cannot stay silent when hour after hour masses of men, women and children are dying or are fleeing destruction and death. The agonising themes of Jew against Muslim, Muslim against Jew must not be exploited as excuses for inhumanity. Before the eyes of the world, humanity on all sides is being reduced to what Shakespeare called poor, bare, forked animals preying on each other like monsters of the deep.

The *New York Times* runs our letter at the top of the letters page, under the headline IMPASSIONED CRIES FROM THE MIDDLE EAST.

A straw in the wind? Who can tell how each action breeds successors and future impulses, changes the climate of the present, if only imperceptibly? Sometimes it can take no more than one straw in the wind. Anyway, we go on waving straws in a world of destruction and rage. Shakespeare knew it in his bones, this near but not total hopelessness: 'How with this rage shall beauty hold a plea / Whose action is no stronger than a flower?'

Back on the domestic front, I'm discovering my duties as an executor of Sadie's will. The two other executors, aware of the smouldering hostility between my brother and sister, warn me that they will withdraw if it flares up into full-scale warfare. More tension. The night before we meet the family accountant, I invite Ruth round for dinner. What begins as a rather wary encounter of two siblings who have not had much contact for years becomes a violent argument about Israel and Lebanon.

I point to my bookshelves. 'You see that section? That's all Judaism – history, prayer-books, Bible, philosophy, jokes, fiction, poems, Holocaust, criticism – it's a kind of soil for me, and it's always changing, always restless, never fixed. And as for being a British Jew – both words are important, British and Jew. I'm a dual person, at least, and so are you, Shakespeare and the English language matter to me as much as the Psalms and Yiddish.'

There's a bit of a silence after that. But she's still not satisfied, must still think I'm something of a traitor. In her eyes my opinions and actions remove me from the flock, make me at best an outsider, at worst an outcast.

We agree to draw a line under this discussion. But I don't want her going away with misconceptions about me, so I say, 'Of course I want Israel to survive, I want the Jews to have a home – the Palestinians too. But to be critical of Israel is not to be disloyal. Criticising

Israel, instead of idolising it, the way in a family you can speak harsh truths about a brother or a sister without breaking off a relationship, may be less blinkered and more helpful.'

She nods at this; am I getting through?

'Maybe not to keep one's mouth shut may almost an obligation for Diaspora Jews. Anyway, I can't live my Jewishness any other way.'

Sunday, August 20, 2006

Barenboim has been holding his annual summer school for the West-Eastern Divan Orchestra, of young Arab and Israeli musicians, which he and Edward Said founded. It takes place in Seville, a city where Jews and Muslims cohabited peacefully and fruitfully, until the Inquisition got to work. There were doubts this year that the school could go ahead at all; young musicians from Arab countries were threatening to boycott an event involving Israelis. Finally, most agreed to come, and the classes and rehearsals went ahead, culminating in a performance of Beethoven's Ninth Symphony in a Seville bull-ring.

The historian Avi Shlaim, coming back from the summer school, tells me how the war bit into Barenboim and his players.

At eleven o'clock at night, after a long day's rehearsal in the heat, Barenboim held up a sheet of paper to the orchestra. 'I have drafted a declaration on behalf of the orchestra,' he said. 'I'm going to read it to you, and then I'd like you to vote for or against by a show of hands.'

The majority were for, but the Israeli contingent was furious about one sentence, referring to the bombing of Lebanese civilians, and proposed a redraft.

They took it to Barenboim next morning. He refused to read it. 'You don't understand,' he said. 'It's too late. Believe me, what I asked you to approve pulls its punches compared to what I would have written had I been speaking on my own behalf, and not the orchestra's.'

The angry Israeli musicians attacked him: 'You're not an Israeli any more. You don't live in the country, you've no idea what we're going through.' Barenboim, who for days had been besieged by reporters, turned his back on them and stormed out.

The orchestra continued its touring engagements. Ten days later, when it was about to appear in Paris, Barenboim wrote in *Le Monde:* 'Time doesn't only affect the content of what we do, it influences it directly. How long will it take for the peoples of the Middle East to accept this fact and to remember that the past is just a transition towards the present, and the present a transition towards the future? So a violent and cruel present will inevitably lead to a violent and cruel future.'

Monday, September 4, 2006

Rosh Hashana Round the Corner.

Bernard Kops, who will be eighty this autumn, writes a rhapsodic review of my biography of Peter Brook in *The Jewish Quarterly*, and I phone him to thank him. 'You ought to use the right-hand side of your brain more,' he said. 'Use your talent to express your own insights, not celebrate the insights of others.'

'How do I do that, Bernard?'

'Come to my playwriting class. Give it a try. If you like it, join.'

So I did, so I do. And witness Bernard's mercurial talent. A dozen writers of varying experience meet weekly in the Kops living room in West Hampstead. Through the French windows (though nothing could be further from the anyone-for-tennis school of drama) comes the sound of excited children playing in the communal garden. Bernard talks, free-associates, performs a playwright's self-communion for this audience. Each term he chooses a classic play to serve as a model, a template. Last year it was Sean O'Casey's *The Shadow of a Gunman*, this year it's Sophocles' *Electra*.

But there's nothing slavish in his use of these texts, nothing academic. He summons them up with the sovereign freedom of a Picasso referencing his forebear Velasquez, loops his way around them, takes them for a walk – as Paul Klee, another sophisticated child-like artist, took a line for a walk. Yet out of these ruminations, we get insights into suspense, turning-points, reversals, revelations – the implements of playwriting.

Some weeks he makes me think he's a modern *Maggid*, in a descent from the inspirational Jewish preachers of eighteenth-century Poland. Many of these Hassidic *rebbes* – men like Jacob Kranz, the Dubner Maggid, famous for his parables, Dov Ber of Mezeritz, disciple of the renowned Baal Shem Tov – became itinerant teachers, creating a tradition of informal, personal, intimate education, which Bernard continues. After Nachman of Bratzlav, Kops of West Hampstead.

He sets us to work. He has prepared a specification for a scene that we are to write in the half-hour leading up to the tea-break. Behind the exercise is the presence of our 'set text', but we are encouraged to play loose and free with it. We buckle down, the room is silent, Bernard busies himself in the kitchen, returns with a big tin of biscuits. Then – and this is the invaluable part of the evening – two actors, who have been invited to join our circle, seize our manuscripts, decipher our handwriting and launch into an immediate performance of our new-hatched scenes. The performance is necessarily sketchy, but a priceless reminder that theatre lives and dies in the instant.

Then everyone comments. Bernard is so quick in his reactions, he seizes the gist of a scene, the ways it might be extended or expanded – or expended. Sometimes his mind is so rapid he reminds me of double doors in a hospital, hinged to open in both directions to allow a trolleyed stretcher to rush through.

Reading his *The World is a Wedding* and *Shalom Bomb*, it's hard not to connect this fluidity of thought and feeling with the mental gates he forced open as a young man, with the nightmares of despair and destruction bred in him by his mother's fearful superstitions and by the annihilation of his Dutch family in the death camps. 'My father had come from Amsterdam, from poverty, and he settled near the docks, like most of the Jews before him, who stayed near the river, I suppose, to keep as close as possible to the Old Country,' he writes in *The World is a Wedding*.

Bernard had to touch bottom before he could resurface, after a long season in hell, like his mentor Rimbaud, fuelled by a reckless regime of drugs – any drugs, in any combination, any substances he could pick up in the nooks and crannies of bohemian post-war Soho.

> The drug had worn off. I was getting the most terrible reaction. Some people call it blowing your top or flipping your lid; only those who have been through it can really know how terrible it is. I left my body. I was a lump of dead flesh spreadeagled over the table, unable to control a single muscle. 'Help.' My long drawn out yell took on a life of its own. I became an empty shell. This, I thought, was the moment of my death. This was the way people went out.

Soho was his refuge from the prison-house of an impoverished home and the neutered suburban aspirations of his relatives. His mother's death triggered his antic disposition, his real madness, his self-induced terror, his fever. These chapters of *The World is a Wedding* rank with the fiercest pages of de Quincey's *Confessions of an English Opium Eater*, Coleridge's *Kubla Khan*, the abysses of Antonin Artaud's *Theatre and its Double*, William Burroughs' dislocated junk world.

No other British Jewish writer has plumbed these depths or felt able to tell the tale, with such vulnerability. Allen Ginsberg has done so, copiously, but that is in another culture, the culture of confession, and it's impossible to imagine the monomaniac American visionary going on to write plays, as Kops has done.

Even in his drug-delirium, Kops did not completely surrender to agony. Grief and dope made him wail and lament, but they didn't stifle his perky humour, the world seen upside down, as Hamlet sees it in his madness. 'I think I understood then what the mad felt. They were really crying out for help but the words got jumbled on the way. I knew what I was trying to say but it all came out different. With astonishment I heard myself utter words unrelated to my thoughts.' Out of these zany dialogues with his doppelgänger, Bernard Kops makes theatre, writes plays.

'As for man, his days are as grass,' laments the funeral service, 'a wind passes over it and it is gone.' Kops at his mother's grave strikes a harsher note:

> I pushed her towards the earth and I covered her with earth. I consigned her to dust. One generation pushes the other into the earth and to make sure the ones we love are out of the way we put them in a box. We feel guilty so we screw the box down. Then we cover this box with earth, then a year later we press a marble stone on top. That's it. Over and done with... As I stood there I thought, 'How beautiful life is, why do we waste so much time?'

One day Bernard rings me. He's just finished a new play, for radio. 'Now I feel exposed,' he says. 'There's nothing between me and the world. As long as I'm writing a play, I'm shielded, I'm safe.'

His plays span fifty years of the British theatre. He began with *The Hamlet of Stepney Green* in 1956, entering a theatre scene cocooned in a post-war eiderdown of reassurance. He blew it away with this play, a song-studded offspring of Shakespeare and Yiddish folk-theatre, an elegy for disappearing Stepney. After its Oxford premiere, it came into the Lyric Hammersmith in 1958, where I saw it at the age of nineteen, and marvelled that Jewish imagination, Jewish humour, Jewish sadness and vitality could be released onto a buttoned-up English stage.

Although British theatre, in the wake of Osborne's *Look Back In Anger* was supposed to be surfing on a revolution, the young Kops wanted to push it further. 'Theatre should be epic, expansive, awash with spectacle, expressionistic and surreal,' he announced, 'but within the matrix of the play there should also be a dynamic to which all could relate. The gods must be driven and affected by the ordinary human stories of tragedy and comedy. They too had their pain, their terrible children who never telephoned them. Social drama, on the other hand, is anathema and best kept for that insatiable god called television. The theatre is the place to take chances.'

British theatre may have unbent somewhat, but it has tended to typecast Kops as a naïve eccentric, a whimsical theatrical Chagall. But as he reaches his four-score, there is a drawing together of threads. He's just finished *Rogues and Vagabonds*, a big play about a travelling troupe of Yiddish actors in 1880s Russia, before the pogroms really got going. All Kops' experience of theatre, from his earliest days as a weekly rep actor feed this Fellini-esque family of laughing, crying, shrewd, quarrelling Yiddish actors. As the troupe's kingly actor-manager affirms:

> We are the Bedouins of nowhere. We exist in a desert of nowhere. Condemned forever to travel through a world of spurious desires. All places, cities, towns, coalesce. The richest and most fortunate people in the world are those who dwell in hovels and live on dreams... We are the holy magicians! We change things. In the middle of nowhere we bring universal theatre. Out of nothing we create something. In the middle of nowhere we create somewhere. We bring life, the muse of

comedy and tragedy! For a brief moment of time, in the middle of *goornicht* we bring certainty, otherness!... We bring transformation. We bring hope.

Autumn 2006

How did I wind up planning to go to India for five weeks?

After sobbing at the sound of Jimmy Rushing's voice, I'd called Peter Brook, and he said, 'I think you might consider putting yourself in a situation you've never been in before. Have you been to India?'

I hadn't. India was an unknown space for me. But I realised after my mother died that I was growing weary of all the things I knew, tired of family routines and political formulae, restless with well-worn words and in general discontented with the familiar. I could see the shape of my thoughts, the colour of my senses, before they arrived. I was settled into my co-ordinates as into a glove. I was ready to learn something new. Putting myself into a *terra incognita* might do the trick.

Brook rang back a few minutes later to suggest I went to see a friend of his, Eduardo, a doctor who lived in London, and was connected to an Ayurvedic clinic in south India. All I knew about Ayurveda was that it was Indian traditional medicine, but I was less inclined than Jane to dismiss it as mumbo-jumbo. 'You should go the clinic in Kerala,' said Peter, 'but I must warn you; it's pretty drastic.' To prepare myself I've been seeing Eduardo. He's Colombian, trained in Western medicine as well as an adept of the Ayurvedic system (his bookshelves are full of Sanskrit texts), every fortnight since being introduced.

There were other, less lofty, reasons why I was keen to try Ayurveda. Weight loss: I was overweight, and couldn't control my urge to eat too much too fast. In fact, the same gobbling had marked my life as a whole; I consumed too many ideas, books, enthusiasms. I didn't give myself time to let any of them take root, just accumulated them.

In one respect, though, my life had begun to change: under the tutelage of Bernard Kops I'd sprung into writing plays – two in fact, one an apprenticeship job, the other in its second draft.

I'd never done this before. For most of my life I had cast myself as a producer, a facilitator and presenter of other people's work. Was I now becoming not so much a producer who occasionally wrote books and scripts, more a playwright who now and then produced performances, documentaries, feature films? Both activities were part of my nature; it was as if the ballast in the ship's hold was shifting.

So 2006 seemed a good moment to go on a course of Indian medicine – Ayurveda, translated in an illustrated manual I am reading, as 'the science, or the wisdom of life', though I ask myself whether the two are the same, and whether 'medicine' is an accurate translation or should it rather be 'healing', and if so, why do I feel uneasy about the New Age, nouveau Californian associations of that word?

A few days before I depart, I go to see the Chola statues at the Royal Academy. Bronze figures of gods and goddesses on plinths, in cases. Their sexual presence, their divine calm: the roundure of breasts, the side-step of weight deflected onto one foot, gently curving the spine, thrusting the hip, angling the haunch. Shiva, multi-armed, dancing, one leg lifted across the body, enclosed in a circle of flames. An aura of dispassionate beauty, impassive power, the work of fine eyes and fingers, still shimmering after ten centuries. They were made for the courts and rulers of the Chola dynasty in southern India, not far from where I'm going. In the exhibition catalogue, the photographer has shot them close-up and cropped, accentuating their eroticism.

The journey is taking on its own structure: twenty-one days in the Ayurvedic clinic in the small Keralan town of Coimbatore, followed by nine days of tourism in the hill stations, tea-plantations, along the backwaters in a long boat; my last few dates in Kochi, which used to be Cochin, the key spice port and site of the last active synagogue in India. I wanted to sit in it and think about my mother. Even venture a prayer or two.

People have been asking me what Ayurvedic medicine is. I tried to imagine it from the illustrated guides I bought in the little India that is Warren Street: being pummelled, becoming isolated, massaged with oils, eating little, getting lighter, purging. I try to explain why I was drawn to it, citing as analogies things I knew, facts of theatre: the alterations in the minds, bodies, voices and imaginations of actors in performance; transformations beyond reason. Jane's brother Tim, a neurologist and a scientific rationalist to his core, listens quietly and says, 'I'm sure it will work, as long as you don't call it medicine.'

That's all right by me. I'm aware of many traditional practices and belief systems that don't fit easily with Western philosophy and science, but have their own reality, as I've seen with Brook when he works with actors from cultures different from our own – African, Vietnamese, Japanese. Or maybe I was gullible. Or just tired of explanations that missed out important aspects of my experience. Jane, even more rationalist and secular than her brother, remains sceptical.

Four days before leaving, I notice pains in my stomach. 'Nerves ahead of the trip?' says Jane. Should I postpone my departure? I ask Eduardo. Although he didn't actually say 'It'll all come out in the wash', Eduardo said that since I was going to a place of healing, it would probably heal my stomach too. I set out for Bombay, and then for a domestic flight south.

Chapter Three:
SUBCONTINENT

Tuesday, March 20, 2007

Arrival in Mumbai.

> Cacophony of klaxons
> Pocked and pitted pavements
> ENGLISH TEACHING CALL-CENTRE TRAINING

> A shrine with a turtle statue at the door
> A man quickly removes his shoes enters
> Touching the door frame then his lips
> Then the turtle

> 'He scored 114 off 87 balls
> And restored the skipper's dogged belief in him'

> A managers' conference
> With flowcharts briefcases lightweight suits
> On 'India Today'

> Three men load a bale of logs
> Onto a bent woman's back
> She staggers
> Past watersellers, Chai brewers, juice vendors
> Slicing ice off a slab with an old plane

Wednesday, March 21, 2007

South to Coimbatore.

My room is about six metres square, and with its well-worn plumbing, iron bed and pavement slab pillows, has the Spartan charm of a monk's cell. Except it's open to the outside world, on one side to a busy little street of small shops – a 'general merchant', a restaurant, 'Veg And Non-Veg', and a baker, where a man spins chappatis on a hot plate all day and into the night. Outside my front door, a cool veranda (it's eleven o'clock, and the temperature still tops the thirties) a big garden, through which a number of pathways converge.

Next morning I sit outside watching women ambling in sandals and young men greeting each other with pinches and touches. The sound of a determined drummer fills the air and through leaves I see candles being lit and the smoke of fires. This must be the temple, I figured, dedicated to Dhanwanthari, the god of healing, whose statues are displayed everywhere.

I have my first consultation with Dilip Kumar, my doctor, a man in his late thirties, with two deferential women assistants. He asks me what's wrong with me. I tell him I have a pain my stomach, stiff knee-joints and want to lose weight. 'You want rejuvenation,' he summarises, dishing out the recipe he must have fed to a thousand patients. 'No no no, that would mean more excitement, not less,' I say; 'I like the age I'm at. I want to empty out my over-full life. I hope to learn to lead a calmer' – not karma, I couldn't resist adding – 'a calmer way of life, less excitable, less full of ideas and things, more quiet for writing.'

He writes it all down on his clipboard.

My breakfast – toast and honey in a tiffin box – arrives and I eat it on the veranda. Mama-figures in *saris* surround me. They look like clinic habitués, once-a-year regular patients. 'Get a life,' I might have said in London.

Our meals are delivered to the room on *thali* trays, with little containers of portions of vegetables, rice or chappatis and a beaker of buttermilk. Diluted buttermilk. I don't feel hungry or miss more substantial dishes for the moment. There must be a lowering of the tide of gastric expectation, a reduction of the stomach's desires.

Like some minor deity, I decide to descend and visit the temple.

Or rather temples, there seem to be a cluster of them, all open to the sky. I am told I must remove my shoes if I wish to enter the precinct. Men and women approach small altars, palms upward in supplication. If they were Jews, they would be asking, 'Almighty, what more do you want of me?' People place their hands palm to palm, lower their heads, murmur quietly. God-effigies crowd under a canopy, garlanded in napkins and flowers.

The hand drummer is getting more syncopated, his voice rising in hoarse invocation. The officiants are male, bare-chested, in their late fifties or more. A couple of men sit together on a platform studying a sacred text, the pupil resting the book open on a lectern, the master barrelling through it at high speed. So much like *yeshivas*.

It's barely seven o'clock and already very hot. I make my way to the library, next to the canteen, serving sugar-free *lassis*, cool and foaming in the heat. The library is two small rooms, sun streaming in. Books on the Ramayana and the hero Arjuna, devout manuals applying ancient teaching to the modern world, share shelfspace with magazines flaunting Bollywood starlets, business management and John Grisham..

I cross a lawn and sit by a giant effigy of P.V. RAMA VARIAR, OUR FOUNDER. BORN ON 24.08.1908 ATTAINED THE LOTUS FEET OF THE LORD ON 10.09.1976. The bust of The Founder is magnified to heroic scale in white plaster, Kim Il Sung style.

In London I'd been reading about Franz Kafka's tuberculosis, much of the latter part of his life spent in Swiss sanatoria. I doubt they were as casually animated as this temple in a clinic.

Saturday, March 24, 2007

1.30am. The third time I've been thrust out of sleep tonight by my rebellious stomach. There's Etna in there, a swirl of gaseous currents and a block of constipation I can't shift. I've never had anything like this. Are these anticipatory symptoms I've induced ahead of the trip? It's been a week since they started. I've followed all the diets and medicines, and tonight it's just got worse.

Prometheus had his liver pecked out for eternity, and Kafka drew out of his punishment one of his most teasing parables.

> There are four legends concerning Prometheus:
> According to the first, he was clamped to a rock in the Caucasus for betraying the secrets of the gods to men, and the gods sent eagles to feed on his liver, which was perpetually renewed.
> According to the second, Prometheus, goaded by the pain of the tearing beaks, pressed himself deeper and deeper into the rock until he became one with it.
> According to the third, his treachery was forgotten in the course of thousands of years, forgotten by the gods, the eagles, forgotten by himself.
> According to the fourth, everyone grew weary of the meaningless affair. The gods grew weary, the eagles grew weary, the wound closed wearily.
> There remained the inexplicable mass of rock. The legend tried to explain the inexplicable. As it came out of the substratum of truth, it had in turn to end in the inexplicable.

I'm following the script and the movement of the myth so far: trying to understand in what ways I have offended that has brought this pain upon me; pressing myself deeper into the pain. Severe stomach cramps for a week – that's all the extent of my suffering. Scarcely Promethean, although inexplicable. But I have at least to describe what's happening. So I haul myself up and write this, eyes gummy, very much the vulnerable ageing man.

Saturday, March 24, 2007

Last night was the big cricket match between India and Sri Lanka. India had to win if she was to stay in the final eight for the World Cup. There's been deafening patriotic drum-beating in *The Times of India,* so I was surprised to find the TV lounge virtually empty as the match began, India bowling. A man came in to wipe the screen clean. He showed us how much gunge had accumulated. He tactfully avoided obscuring play itself, not so hard when Rupert Murdoch's Star TV peppers the match with ad breaks.

India takes a couple of wickets in the first half hour, then it settles into a war of attrition. Members of the clinic's staff creep in to watch. Two phlegmatic men of immense girth plump down in the front row, and talk throughout, one channel-hopping to a match from another group. I'm irritated and slope off to bed, wake later to see that Sri Lanka have won. Scenes of national desolation.

In the *New York Times,* Shashi Tharoor asks why cricket has never taken on in America, though baseball, its simplified cousin, has:

> Cricket was better suited to a country like India, where a majority of the population still consults astrologers and believes in the capricious influence of the planets — so they can well appreciate a sport in which, even more than in baseball, an ill-timed cloudburst, a badly prepared pitch, a lost toss of the coin

at the start of a match or the sun in the eyes of a fielder can transform the outcome of a game. Even the possibility that five tense, hotly contested, occasionally meandering days of cricket-ing could still end in a draw seems derived from ancient Indian philosophy, which accepts profoundly that in life the journey was as important as the destination. Not exactly the American Dream.

None of these beliefs, I fear, will be much consolation to these Indian fans.

The Times of India Sunday edition reports the death at 89 of U G Krishnamurti, far removed from the stereotype of the mystical, spiritual Indian. U G Krishnamurti defied all classifications – a philosopher, a non-guru or guru, he was described as 'subversive, revolutionary and totally fearless'. UG blasted all spiritual discourses as 'poppycock' and thrashed spiritual masters as 'misguided fools'.

'A messiah is one who leaves a mess behind him in the world.' 'Religions have promised roses, but all you end up with are the thorns' – quotable one-liners from UG, who also detested being called an enlightened man. 'I can't find any other way to describe the way I am functioning,' he would say. 'At the same time I would point out there is no such thing as enlightenment.' UG rejected the notion of soul or *atman* and declared that our search for permanence was the cause of our suffering. He lectured to the Theosophical Society, where he met his more famous namesake, J Krishnamurti, but he later rejected JK's philosophy, calling it 'a bogus chartered journey'.

He moved to America with his family for medical treatment of his son's polio, and took lectures to American audience to pay for medical expenses. After two years he lost interest in lecturing and his marriage of seventeen years ended. After aimless wanderings in London and Paris, he wound up in Geneva and lived in the chalet of a rich follower.

On his forty-ninth birthday and for seven days afterwards, reports *The Times of India*, he underwent a 'clinical death'. Seven bewildering physical changes took place, and he landed in what he called the 'natural state'. 'He would say he had no "message for mankind", but thousands the world over would flock to listen to his 'anti-teaching.'

I will have to reassure Jane I did not make up this man, so much she would admire his uncompromising positions.

In the agony column of the same newspaper:

> *My husband has developed a strange fetish. Every time we have sex, he insists on playing Alfred Hitchcock–style suspense movie music at a very loud volume. What does this signify?*
>
> *Unless he asks you to step into the shower [writes the agony aunt], I think you can rest in peace that it is just a harmless diversion.*

Sunday, March 25, 2007

First massage, with warm oil. The treatment room reminds me of Abu Ghraib. Dull grey-green institutional walls. Rope hanging from hook in the ceiling. And dominating the room, a chunky wooden treatment slab. Its funnels disperse the oil from the surface, which soon becomes as slippery as a skating rink. In Abu Ghraib, it was blood.

My masseur Shijith, a thin wiry young man, takes off his shirt, rolls up his trouser legs, and starts. A stream of warm oil hits my head, which he rubs and shakes. Oil from plants, to judge by the leaves on the bottle label. Soon I'm drenched in it, as he works his way along every limb and joint. When he asks me to turn over, I'm skidding across the oiled surface and he's stopping me falling off.

It lasts an hour, and it's not unpleasant. The thought of being covered in oil was worse than the experience. Shijith runs hot water into a barrel, opens a bag of white powder, mixes it with water into a paste. 'What's that?' I ask.

'Moon powder' was what his answer sounds like, so 'moon powder' shall be what it becomes. I find out later it's mung powder, made of mung beans. He scrubs my skin with moonpaste and pours jugs of hot water over me.

When I emerge, feeling scrubbed, stretched and pummelled, I meet Ulrike, a Viennese-born woman who has retired from working as a clinic administrator in Harley Street. 'How well do think this place is managed?' I ask. 'This place? It's Fawlty Towers,' she says, 'but it works.' I ask her why she's here – I'm beginning to fall into the communal subtext of asking about symptoms and progress. She comes for lower back pain, she says. 'Five weeks every two years and my back's good for another two years,' she says. 'I have seen people who had to be carried in walk out of here unaided. But I have never seen miracle cures for weight loss.' Jane will find this a touch dispiriting, but we shall see. I get Jitesh to fit me a broadband connection in my room. Now I'm in touch with Jane and the world of friends.

For the past few days, I've been eating honey and toast, south Indian vegetables with rice cakes or chappatis, buttermilk, water. If it's true that all the toxins in my body are being emptied out – into my lower intestine? – then the digestion gets weaker, and these lean rations are probably the most it can handle.

Enough symptomology. I don't want to turn into a modern *malade imaginaire*, whose hypochondriac hero obsessively scrutinises the contents of his chamber-pot, while tyrannising over everyone in his household, except doctors, who he reveres.

Molière: such comic energy, such clarity of structure, such symmetry of plot and payoff. *Le Malade Imaginaire* was his last play. He understood doctors and medicine; he'd been ill himself. He played Argan, the protagonist, sitting in a grand chair, half throne, half commode. He wasn't feeling well during the first three performances, but no one in his company took much notice of that; the boss was always complaining. During the fourth performance, he had an attack and died on stage.

But before this positively final appearance, he must have enjoyed playing the exchanges between Argan and Toinette, his devoted servant and sharpest critic. In Scene Eight, she enters disguised as a doctor.

> TOINETTE: Give me your pulse. (*To pulse.*) Come, behave yourself: beat the way you're meant to. I'll show you the way to behave, make no mistake. Hah, this pulse is playing the upstart with me. (*To pulse.*) I see you haven't begun to know who you're dealing with yet. Who was your doctor?
>
> ARGAN: Monsieur Purge Me.
>
> TOINETTE: Not on my register of qualified doctors. Where does he say your illness comes from?
>
> ARGAN: He says it's from the liver. Others say, the spleen.
>
> TOINETTE: Ignoramuses, the lot of them! What you're suffering from is the lung.
>
> ARGAN: The lung?
>
> TOINETTE: Yes. What do you feel?
>
> ARGAN: Now and then I get headaches.
>
> TOINETTE: Exactly, the lung.
>
> ARGAN: Sometimes I seem to have a veil before my eyes.
>
> TOINETTE: The lung.
>
> ARGAN: Then a kind of lassitude creeps through all my limbs.
>
> TOINETTE: The lung.
>
> ARGAN: And sometimes I get stomach cramps. Like colic.
>
> TOINETTE: The lung. Do you have a good appetite?
>
> ARGAN: Yes, Monsieur.

TOINETTE: The lung. Do you like having a glass or two of wine?

ARGAN: Yes, Monsieur.

TOINETTE: The lung. After the meal you need a little nap, and you sleep deeply?

ARGAN: Yes, Monsieur.

TOINETTE: The lung. The lung, I'm telling you.

(Translated by Michael Kustow)

...and I leave Molière's satire on medical credulity there, just before he hits comic top gear by making his doctor prescribe that the patient should dig out an eye and cut off an arm because they are leaching sustenance from the other side of the body. This tests even the *malade imaginaire*'s credulity. No playwright knew better than Molière that in every clinic and sanatorium – as in every religion and party – there are the dependent, the devotees and the cynical exploiters.

Monday, March 26, 2007

Sweet-smelling clouds roll down the corridors, from a plant-pot of incense carried by a young man, his dusk duty.

I have just come out of my third massage. Jitesh the masseur said a prayer under his breath before he began, and was not too brutal. It's switch slide slip sideways in oil infused with herbal decoctions, heated, cooled, heated and cooled again, twelve times before it's let out. At the end, he brings a palm full of brown powder, rubs it into my head – I'm too slow to stop him – and holds it to my nose to inhale. Sandalwood.

He reminds me of the Mohican-haircut, loincloth-wearing, bare-buttocked actor I saw at the Roundhouse just before I left: a punk Puck in Tim Supple's *Midsummer Night's Dream*. Or more recently, the absurd posing oiled and muscled actors playing Spartans fighting the Persian army in the lamentable epic *300* which I saw in a Mumbai suburb, because I was too late to get into the Bollywood film I was after.

Writing about *300* in *The Guardian* Peter Bradshaw reports that:

> the political and media classes of Iran are reportedly up in arms about this fantastically silly retelling of the Battle of Thermopylae in 480BC... With the kind of tremulous fervour that only pre-pubescent boys can work up on the subject of war, it recounts how the barbarous invading hordes of Persia were heroically held back by just 300 oiled and muscly Spartan warriors long enough for the Greek armies to regroup and for Athenian democracy – and by implication, all our inherited western values – to be saved for ever more. Iranian commentators, sudden and quick in quarrel, have found the slight intolerable. These people will presumably now redouble their commitment to historical sensitivity with another Holocaust Denial Conference.

Sometimes I think I consume too much journalism, too many hasty opinions. But when journalists are this spiky and irascible, who can resist?

Much more offensive to the Iranians than the idealisation of the handful of plucky Spartans should have been a truly lifeless performance as the Persian king Xerxes by another male model with campy body language and perfect pecs. But a poor actor in a posing pouch should not be a reason to start a war between Iran and the West.

Tuesday, March 27, 2007

One thing I like about this Fawlty Towers of a clinic is the number of capable women in good jobs. Parvati, a calm woman in her fifties, commands the front desk. Dr Shendil Rani, one of my medical doctors, very serious, won't borrow my copy of Arundhati Roy's novel *The God of Small Things* until she knows she'll have time to read it. One of my daily doctors is a woman, Dr Rani. She seemed at first a little severe, as if determined not to smile until she knew me better. Now she does, and laughs when I make jokes. Tall Dr Rohani, an analyst from the research institute, comes in to check my reflexes with the customary little rubber hammer. Women do blood tests, take pulse-beats, but that's not so different from at home.

But the three dark and gleeful women who clean the rooms and landings would stand out anywhere. Three tall, infectiously giggling graces wearing bright green overalls, their long braided hair hanging like bell-pulls; there's nothing craven about them. Pointing to their identity tags, they tell me their names: V Kamalaveni (a tall woman with a spine like a column, who has two children in their twenties); P Umarani (lots of gold-leaf markings and ear-rings, three children); K Vasanthi (the youngest, two children).

They might be from a lower caste, but no one will tell me. Like all women here, they wear sandals, and glide, rather than clop pavements. Maybe I like that because there's something Old Testament about it: Ruth carrying a pitcher of water from the well. They speak a little English, but can't read it. Maybe what I call Old Testament is just shorthand for poor, un-educated village life.

They notice the screensaver on my computer, a dissolving sequence of Rembrandt self-portraits. I try to explain who Rembrandt is. They look at his face, morphing from bright young dandy with an earring to the weight and stillness of age. Three young women watching a life-cycle on a Toshiba screen.

Wednesday, March 28, 2007

My first venture out on the street since I arrived.

An ox with horns painted bright green, tethered to shafts of a cart. A heavily-built woman butcher, wielding an axe on the carcass of a lamb. An almost as burly woman fruit vendor slicing the tops off coconuts with a sickle. Painted plasterwork temples – Krishna, Shiva and his full-bosomed partner, Parvati. A building with a partially-hidden elephant sign which sounds promising. No such luck. On closer inspection, it's 'Ganesh Astrological Centre'.

Garlands of flowers, which women wear round necks or hair, and I buy for the room, white and orange. Above all, little shops. Coimbatore, like many Indian towns, is a nest of small retailers. One-storey shopfronts spilling onto the pavement, selling clothes, international telephone cards and above all food – cheap, plentiful, straight from the farm. Old women squat in the dust next to heaps of green bananas. Big men in small kiosk windows shout to the passers-by, promising unimaginable bargains.

I know this world, its street theatre, its slogans, its superlatives. I'm the son of a small retailer.

Thursday, March 29, 2007

I'm still not sleeping because of the stomach spasms. I wander off at daybreak in search of people to talk to, even though I hardly managed to sleep for more than half-hour bursts.

Giancarlo, born in Scotland from a family of Italian immigrants, lives in Peru with a Venezuelan wife, and produces world music discs and films. Giancarlo is a friend of Eduardo, my Colombian-born Ayurvedic physician. He turns out to have, thankfully, a good sense of humour about his ancestors. We laugh at the picture of his great-grandfather from Civitavecchia trying to sell ice-cream from a handcart in Dundee during a snowstorm.

In the computer room, I meet Didier, a classic French type – the *louche* disarray of a Serge Gainsbourg, the fluent, 100 kilometre-an-hour speech and offhand body language of a Belmondo. Like Giancarlo, he too was in the music business, though at the more experimental end of rock, it seems, including its addiction to alcohol and drugs. I take pleasure in dusting out the vernacular French I learned as a member of a French theatre troupe fifty years ago; he seems pleased to have found a Francophile Englishman.

We stand in the courtyard, watching women in *saris* glide past. I say I find the way they walk with their pelvis thrust forward kind of erotic. 'India's the least erotic place I know,' pronounces Didier with all the sexual certitude of a Frenchman. 'Nothing turns me on – and I'm not a hard man to get going.'

Friday, March 30, 2007

Week one of my three is over. Week two, the climactic one, is for *Panchakarma*, the most intensive treatment. I have put on Celia's wrap-around *lunghi* as I scurry to my first intensive treatment, The Big Purification. Haven't worn anything this skirt-like since I was told to cover up my legs in Jerusalem on the Temple Mount. Outside the Al Aqsa Mosque, I looked silly, but kind of fetching as well.

This session will involve six pairs of hands on me at once. My Ayurvedic manual also talks alarmingly about purges and enemas. Giancarlo is sitting outside his room, looking relaxed and exhausted. 'Had your treatment, Giancarlo?' He nods. 'How was it?' Pause, as if he's trying to sort out how it was. 'A trip.'

The treatment room is crowded – six people, each with a segment of me to service on the slab, and one to draw liquid calligraphies on my head.

The rope which has been dangling above my head now holds a big bowl of unheated oil which, as I lie down, drools down onto my head through a tassel poking through its bottom. I knew there had to be use for it, and am glad it's not torture.

No fewer than six masseurs work over my body with the warm oil, while a seventh dribble pencils of cool oil across my forehead.

After forty minutes, I get restless, and start singing. I give them *Summertime* – why not? – and ask one of them to sing a song back in Tamil or Malayalam. General embarrassment: maybe it's too sacred a ritual to sing in, maybe the boy's afraid of being laughed at by his mates.

I float, I merge. It's like being licked by the smooth tongues of eager puppies. Not better than sex, but better than some sex I can remember.

The theory is that the toxins will now be mobilised by the hot oil/cold oil treatment, which will open up the pores and put the waste matter in my intestines. When it's over, we're not allowed now to go out any further than the veranda; the immune system being very weak, we must be sheltered.

Saturday, March 31, 2007

Gastric War: after weeks of skirmishes and delusive victories, an inner monsoon hits my belly in the early hours, flushing away its contents (and what feels like some intestinal lining) and leaving me dehydrated, weak as a mouse and a happier man. It feels like the purge to end all purges.

I am wrong. It's not over yet.

The Tamil Tigers, who want an independent state for Tamils, pull off a daring sortie and for the first time bomb a Sri Lankan military base, which frightens everyone.

The Hindu regrets that countries like Russia, China, France and Germany, knowing the way the wind is blowing, have seen fit to appease American policy again. 'The irony is that each believed it was moderating Washington's agenda whereas it was actually Washington that was getting its script enacted.'

They don't even mention Britain. We're written out of the equation from the start. I glimpse Tony Blair on the television news, still grinning boyishly. He reminds me of that sketch by the great French mime Marcel Marceau, *The Mask-Maker,* in which the actor contorts his face as he adopts a succession of masks, and then finds he can't remove the last one. It's become a fixture of his face. Blair's like that. But so are most politicians. Like bad actors, they are marketing a known brand image.

My doctor in London e-mails asking what effects the intensive *Panchakarma* is having on my mind and body. My stomach pains wake me at 1.30am, and I reply:

Dear Eduardo,

As I start these notes on the effect of the *Panchakarma* on my body, I fear you are going to be very disappointed in me.

It seems to me that the true harvest of what I have been doing/what has been done to me has been almost wiped out by the effects of my stomach infection.

To be blunt, I have not had one uninterrupted night's sleep since I arrived here two weeks ago. If you add on the week before that when as you know I was suffering from a stomach infection in London and could not sleep either, this means that for three weeks I have not had unbroken sleep.

This does not give me a good vantage point to report to you on the physical changes and benefit of the treatment here, let alone any spiritual insights.

I have had to spend hours in the waking day catching up on my sleep, rather than following the effects of the treatments. I have nonetheless noted the first impact of the oils, the massage, the diet. A great simplification has been at work. If it were not for my skirmishes with the effects of constipation and diarrhoea (I have called it the First Gastric War), I would be able to report in more detail. But you need to have a functioning bodily instrument to do so.

I feel a great sense of waste to have come all this way, made these preparations with you, only to have the results spoiled by this belly-aggression, these testy bowels and this gastric waste.

On some days, when equilibrium has been restored and sleep to some extent regained, I have experienced a clearer picture of my body and its distinct functions, a body-map which I will retain.

Maybe I have idealised my expectations of the results of Ayurveda on the whole of my organism.

I have not been able to slow down my mind and evacuate its contents, though I feel I have more mental space available and that it is less cluttered.

It's also certain that without this laptop I would have felt even more wretched. Writing what's been happening is also a physical/mental response.

The *Pizhichil* and *Dhara* have had a soothing and wonderfully...musical effect. A glimpse of my flesh as a delight and a continual metamorphosis. Now that this phase of treatment is over, I will miss it. I may even miss the fast and purge which ended it – what I called the Mass Evacuation. It left me wiped out, exhausted, but not unhappy.

This is all I can offer you this morning (1.15am) in reply to your question.

Sunday, April 1, 2007

I think of the young doctor Chekhov and all his talents as I talk to my young doctors. Their mentor, Dr Keshavan, Senior Medical Officer, tells me he won a scholarship to film school, wanted to be a director, but his father insisted he studied medicine. Remind me of anyone?

I've been up since six, sitting with Giancarlo, looking into the courtyard. It's quiet and almost empty.

A man sweeps leaves with a broom, not a gesture too much, taking his time.

Water-bearers carry big pitchers of medicated water to the treatment rooms.

The women walk past in *saris*, with an unhurried, undulating step. The way a *sari* hangs: one long white piece of cloth interfolded and easily worn.

The sun is just starting to come up, and almost orange against the leaves and red blossom.

A young woman squats and draws a flower circle on the flagstones, drizzling coloured dust. A pavement artist chalking her first mandala of the morning.

When Peter Brook said that he thought I should try something quite different in my life, he had already thrown me the net of P D Ouspensky's book on Gurdjieff, *In Search of The Miraculous*, giving it to me as a first-night present in 1966. I did not take the bait. Now he's made a second attempt by getting me to come here. He might have been saying, after my mother's death, 'Follow my example, and take yourself in hand.' Gurdjieff applies 'shocks' to stop us in our tracks, take a real look at what, who and where we are, and face the possibility of change.

Peter is one of the father figures, the elders, whom I elected in the first part of my life as role models. He embodies many qualities

I would like to have: he's cosmopolitan, he leads a theatre company; he's alert to paradox. Other elders have stood for other qualities: Shaike Weinberg for socialism and scepticism; David Perlov for the poetic gaze of his camera lens; David Sylvester for his gravity and his carved prose.

The process of writing Brook's biography over three years could have undermined our friendship. Instead, I think it's deepened it, and levelled the playing field between us. I no longer feel so much like his son. But I pay attention to his most offhand word, and that's why it's he who has catapulted me into India.

The outside world thrusts in. A cockroach with ten legs crawls its way out of the plug-hole. Killing it is like trying to kill Jack Nicholson in Kubrick's *The Shining*; it refuses to die and keeps on coming. I finish it off with the base of a tin mug.

Monday, April 2, 2007

The guerrilla warfare in my nether regions continues. Puffs of gunfire puncture my bellyspace. Has this Gastric War in my gut reduced me to a foretaste of what I may be as an old man? My time in Coimbatore is nearly up. Am I about to leave this refuge feeling not much better than when I arrived?

I make a little anthology of remembered lines about ageing and final departures.

> Time held me green and dying
>
> *Dylan Thomas, 'Fern Hill'*

> An agèd man is but a paltry thing,
> A tattered coat upon a stick, unless
> Soul clap its hands and sing, and louder sing
> For every tatter in its mortal dress
>
> *W B Yeats, 'Sailing to Byzantium'*

In me thou see'st the glowing of such fire,
That on the ashes of his youth doth lie,
As the death-bed, whereon it must expire,
Consumed with that which it was nourish'd by.

Shakespeare, Sonnet 73

(Shakespeare's characteristic fascination with opposites – how the best can turn into the worst, how what sustains you can also kill you. Anti-cancer drugs can work like this.)

EARL OF GLOUCESTER: O, let me kiss that hand!

LEAR: Let me wipe it first; it smells of mortality.

Shakespeare, 'King Lear'

(Was Shakespeare remembering the smell of shit on his hand?)

Now it is autumn and the falling fruit
and the long journey towards oblivion.

The apples falling like great drops of dew
to bruise themselves an exit from themselves...

Already our bodies are fallen, bruised, badly bruised,
already our souls are oozing through the exit
of the cruel bruise.

Already the dark and endless ocean of the end
is washing in through the breaches of our wounds,
Already the flood is upon us.

Oh build your ship of death, your little ark
and furnish it with food, with little cakes, and wine
for the dark flight down oblivion.

D H Lawrence, 'The Ship of Death'

'Pain,?' says the man on the cool oil, as I groan and shift. 'Pain? Pain?' What I feel is not the pain of those in Zimmer frames or wheelchairs, but it's pain okay, pain and danger. It could at best be described as sleep-murdering discomfort, but I can't say that. So I say, 'Pain.' And he seems content with my reply.

Will I ever be able to trust my solar plexus again? I feel a radical insecurity at my centre. Am I softened up enough to become a fall guy for things esoteric?

The sociological, the historical, the political, and the psychological: I can hear their reasoning coming a long way off. I came to India looking for something in addition. I came to India not as a devotee or adept, but because at a critical moment just after my mother's death it seemed the right thing to do. Even if I could not anticipate the rocky road it became.

I hear the voice of my cool-oil masseur: 'Pain. Pain. Pain.'

Diagnostic techniques unchanged since my childhood. Tongue stuck out, sharp intake of breath, head shaking in dismay. 'Coated.'

Pulse. Ear, nose, throat. Blood pressure. Morning motion.

When the maps and explanations of new science take over, what happens to the old maps and metaphors, used for centuries?

Like everything in India, Ayurveda was built on categorisations. To Earth, Air, Fire and Water, Ayurveda adds Ether, and maps these five elements across to the five human senses. Psyche, body and cosmos connect, as in Elizabethan 'humours': sanguine, choleric, phlegmatic, melancholic.

No one's a hundred per cent one or the other. I guess I'm melancholic/choleric.

In Ayurveda, there are three clusters of bio-energy, indicating three basic human types, *vata*, *pitta* and *kapha*. When these three are in balance, you're fine. Out of balance, you're in trouble.

I came to Coimbatore because, like Hamlet's time, I was 'out of joint'. I half-knew this before I left England. But I couldn't see a way to re-balance it in London.

Tuesday, April 3, 2007

Outside the television room I say hello to Maya, a tall, fortyish woman from Russia. She's here with her even taller (pushing seven foot) son, Mikhail, a gangling distracted young man who can't look at anyone when he speaks to them and is said to be suffering from an attention deficit syndrome called Internet Addiction. He's just told the doctor he won't continue taking treatment if he's not allowed to watch television whenever he wants to. He comes out, stooping so as to avoid the doorframe, followed by his doctor, who reaches about as far as his elbow.

I wonder what Krishna Kumar would do to help Mikhail. Krishna Kumar is the Managing Director of the cluster of companies that make up this Ayurvedic enterprise. Seated behind a desk packed with papers and mementos, he has a big, leonine head, a gaze that rivets you with its unmoving attention. Attention Plenitude Syndrome, perhaps.

We talk about the dependency of the patient on the doctor; religion practised merely as outward observance which only fosters dependent thinking; the dumbing-down of Indian education. It's not so much what we said that I remember, it's his gaze, his focus, his stillness. He has founded a school, and is starting another, to teach quality, and not just factual quantity – anyway, that's my definition.

'Do you have to be rich to afford to go to your schools?' I ask. 'No,' he says. 'I fund them out of donations to the temple.'

Unable to bide my peace, unable to accept simply being a patient, I suggest to him that I do a Shakespeare workshop as a benefit for the clinic before I leave, taking sonnets and speeches and scenes and working on them with local actors in front of an audience. Krishna says that although there is no theatre in Coimbatore, he will have no difficulty in finding performers, even if they are not professionals: 'Indian people love Shakespeare.'

I shouldn't be doing this, I'm meant to be taking things in, not putting them out, but I can't resist. The side of me that is a producer, a performer – and yes, a narcissist who rises to an audience – is too strong. The bustling side of me that wants to make things happen in the three-dimensional world, not just on paper, won't lie down.

I learned about Shakespeare from years watching and listening as a member of Peter Hall's Royal Shakespeare Company in the early 1960s. And above all I learned my way about Shakespeare from another key elder in my life, John Barton. Peter Hall had plucked John from King's College Cambridge, where he was an eccentric and much-loved English don and a leading light in university theatre as actor, director and adaptor of classic texts. John's feeling for Shakespearean verse, and his mastery of the simplest, most direct communication techniques embedded in that verse, stamped the first generation of the RSC with an indelible and flexible style. Gone were the noble flutings of yesteryear; but equally gone was the sleeves-rolled-up iconoclasm of the new wave of actors, shaped by Royal Court vernacular drama and the naturalism of screen acting.

John taught ways of letting 'poetry' arise out of obedience to the rules of Shakespearean verse – antithesis, setting one word against another; observing line endings; above all, not being appalled by a lengthy wad of text in blank verse. He's a wonderful teacher and guide because he's lovable and eccentrically attractive in himself. He has authority, but exerts it in a series of modest suggestions to the actor. Blessed with a sharp-featured face that could come out of an Elizabethan miniature, chomping anti-smoking gum, roaming around the stage completely oblivious to his environment (chairs and coffee-cups tumbled in his path; once, eagerly making a point, he walked backwards off the edge of stage and fell into the front row of the stalls but never stopped talking), John had given the fledgling RSC acting company a coherence, a basis from which they could soar.

In the 'eighties, I commissioned a television series of John's Shakespeare workshops; seeing him take the likes of Judi Dench, Sinead Cusack, Susan Fleetwood, Sheila Hancock, Alan Howard, Ben Kingsley, Jane Lapotaire,

Ian McKellen, Michael Pennington, Roger Rees, Patrick Stewart and David Suchet – a whole generation of actors – lodged itself in my mind as a touchstone of language in theatre.

Now, in southern India, the pupil that I was takes on the role of the workshop master, in a rudimentary hall next to the temple on the clinic campus. I sent Krishna Kumar my curriculum vitae and the copy for a leaflet, and asked him to choose performers for me. In reply, I get an effusive, not to say blush-making, response: 'Respected Michaelji, Namaste! I am so happy that I met a living legend like you.' He asks me for my birth date and time, to read my horoscope.

He sets about finding me actors. Since there's no theatre in Coimbatore, he chooses students and teachers: two seventeen-year-old girls and their aunt, and a relative who taught Shakespeare and Eng Lit in Indian schools, and who had lately lost her husband to leukaemia. They look like an interesting bunch, but we don't have a single male in the cast.

With only twenty-four hours to go, the phone in my room rings.

'I gather you are looking for people to perform Shakespeare extracts,' says a percussive, forthright, male voice. 'I may be able to help you. I've done a bit of acting and I love Shakespeare. I'm downstairs at reception. Would you like to meet?'

Waiting for me downstairs is a short man with a ramrod spine, bristling with energy like a coiled spring. I ask him his name.

'Matthews.'

'And your first name?'

'Major Mathews,' he replies fiercely.

'But don't you have a first name?'

'Major is my first name. I was an officer in the Indian army, where we did some Shakespeare. Now I am retired.'

For Major Matthews, that concludes the interview. He wants to get down to work, show me what he can do. I handed him a page with Hamlet's 'To be or not to be' on it. We're going in at the deep end. I ask him to try it. He begins, reeling out the lines as if they were orders from a commanding office. I stop him.

'Let's try a couple of simple things, Major. This speech is a soliloquy. Not a monologue, a soliloquy. The character – and the actor – is conscious of the presence of an audience. Imagine I'm the audience. Can you try it line by line, checking after each one to see whether you are getting through to me?'

He does so; it's slower and shapelier, directed towards listeners, a big improvement.

'Now let's try something else. Notice how many questions there are in this speech? Hamlet is desperately seeking an answer to all the questions besieging him – who would bear the whips and scorns of time, who would these fardels bear?... He wants answers, and he knows there's an audience with him there in the room. So use this audience. Ask them the questions. Insist on replies. You can improvise between Shakespeare's lines.'

He does so – 'Now you in the second row, give me an answer'; 'Nobody leaves this room until I've got some answers'; 'Why are we all so resigned, such cowards, tell, tell me!' He's a Shakespearean major now, berating his hapless platoon, throwing himself angrily at the text, like a champion batsman hitting sixes. Parade-ground Shakespeare perhaps, but the text comes alive.

About fifty people turn up for the workshop itself next day; most of the doctors and nurses have gone to a rival meeting, a religious dissertation. I am invited to light a candle at a shrine by the side of the stage, to bless our event. First come the two students, to whom I've given Shakespeare sonnets. What they do is terrible – sing-song, sugary, dutiful, nursery recitation, as if Shakespeare were A A Milne.

'But that's how we've been taught,' they protest. I realise they're at the fag end of a long line of 'Shakespeare elocution' in India, stretching back to the early nineteenth century, when speaking Shakespeare was part of the entry exams to the Indian Civil Service. The ancestors of these young women were schooled in that tradition, taught to deliver Shakespeare's verse 'musically', with the reverence due to a Sacred Genius imported by the British. Unwittingly, I've bumped into one of the last cultural vestiges of colonialism.

I lay into the young women, perhaps too fiercely; Anjolie, one of India's leading painters, who has come here to cure a back pain she got dancing salsa too vigorously, is watching and later tells me I made the mistake of criticising Indian students in public. 'You overlooked their *amour propre*.'

But I manage to jolt them out of the iambic hypnotic spell, and into some semblance of love, anxiety, desire, hope – the real things that the Sonnets express. At least I manage to dispel some of the gentility in which their Shakespeare has been swathed.

It's time for Major Matthews to make his assault on 'To be or not to be'. He hurls himself at it, and now that we have an actual audience, buttonholes individuals, using his own improvised words between Shakespeare's: '"The law's delay" – come on now, why should you put up with these law wallahs keeping you waiting?' '"The insolence of office" – who are these jumped-up mediocrities pushing you around? Don't put up with it!' I find myself applauding his vehemence as he fillets Shakespeare's text with his own insertions. After the colonial sing-song, this comes alive.

The final performer is the newly widowed handsome woman. In our rehearsals, I'd hardly had to give her a note, she connected her own rage with Lady Macbeth's scorn for her lily-livered husband and her denatured ambition to kill Duncan and seize the throne. Now she launches into one of Shakespeare's most hair-raising speeches with burning fury:

> I have given suck, and know
> How tender 'twas to love the babe that milks me;
> I would, while it was smiling in my face,
> Have plucked my nipple from his boneless gums
> And dash'd the brains out, had I so sworn as you
> Have done to this.

She finds a violence which is almost frightening in the form as well as the content of these lines. Working on Lady Macbeth's ruthless speech reminds me of the fear of death and separation in the Sonnets. With the loss of her husband, maybe her awareness of the irreversibility of death is sharpened. But there's something more. When she calls on the spirits to 'unsex me here,' she denatures her femininity with the often frenzied violence with which the history of the subcontinent is spattered. This is a Shakespeare who is naked, brutal, and aware that all limits are fragile. It's light-years away from the traditional veneration for Shakespeare in India.

Tuesday, April 10, 2007

Goodbye, India. Goodbye, Coimbatore. Goodbye, *saris* and sandals, mandalas and shrines. Goodbye, clinic companions. I don't know whether I'll see you again. I am leaving the clinic, after three weeks' treatment, which may have done me good but has failed to remove the pain in my stomach or correct the lurching walk – shuffle, rather – which I've developed in the past few days. I called Eduardo in London, but he screamed that I was interrupting a session with another patient, and that his mother was dying in Colombia. 'Do you not have any consideration for the plight of others?'

I have decided to truncate the ten-day tourist trip I had booked, and have asked the travel agent to find me a ticket home sooner. It's insane for me to go sightseeing and floating along the backwaters of Kerala when Jane's in England and I feel like shit. If I never come back, India will forever seem like unfinished business.

An old saloon car draws up in the courtyard, and I bid farewell to my hosts and fellow patients, truth-seekers, inmates. We head up to the hills, to the tea plantations and cooler, autumnal temperatures. My stomach is as tender as a retina, and shaken by the hairpin bends and bumpy roads. I try lying down across the back seat, but it's worse, so I console myself by enjoying the rocks and peaks all round. We arrive at Munnar, go through another busy market place and up, to a hillside settlement of bungalows. I step out, into a fine spume of mist and drizzle, welcome after the heavy heat of the clinic. For two days, I sleep, eat and hobble along the hill path, looking down on toy houses in the deep valley. On the third day, we drive to Kochi, my final destination, and the site of the last remaining synagogue in India.

On a bright, windy Saturday the driver takes me to 'Jewtown' (Kochi had no inhibitions about naming its neighbourhoods) and to the synagogue. An airy room built by the Portuguese Jewish settlers in the seventeenth century, it's floored in blue Delft tiles. Gauzy curtains blow in from lofty windows. There are half a dozen old men in the *shul* for the Shabbat morning service. I sit and look at the prayer-book. I wander around in the space to different positions. I think about my mother.

I'm not feeling too good, though, and decline the invitation to help make up a *minyan*. On the drive back to Kochi, the driver babbles on about Dan Brown and his *Da Vinci Code*, which has been published in India, and which has sown doubt in the heart of my driver. I'm depressed that the cult of this bestseller has reached Hindus in Southern India. None of my attempts to demystify it make much difference to the driver. I spend a night in a ridiculously plush business-person's hotel (India racing into modernity) and next morning he drives me to the airport to fly to Colombo in Sri Lanka, from where I fly to London. It's an unsatisfactory departure. I feel let down. I was meant to be in the hands of doctors, admittedly of another medical persuasion, and they not only failed to treat the waves of pain in my stomach, which were stopping me sleeping, but also discharged a man visibly ill.

I take with me a little bronze Ganesha, and try to adopt its amused equanimity.

Chapter Four:
HOMECOMING

Sunday, April 15, 2007

London.

I arrive at London Heathrow after an eleven-hour journey via Sri Lanka – all tickets via Mumbai were sold out, I had to fly south to Colombo to get a plane to fly north to England. I am not in good shape, find it hard to walk in a straight line. I get onto the Heathrow Express. After one station, the train stops and a nasal loudspeaker voice says, 'This train goes no further. Please continue your journey on the following train.' I stumble out, and as the train draws away, realise I have left my luggage on it. Not the most auspicious of arrivals. I weave my way unsteadily to the Lost Property counter, and explain what has happened. But the words don't seem to be coming out in the right order.

> Me and my shadow
> Strolling down the avenue
> Me and my shadow
> All along and feeling kind of blue…

My dad used to sing this Flanagan and Allen song, which comes into my mind as I climb the stairs and Jane opens the door to me. Her jaw drops. The man who left her in tolerable human repair returns as a confused shambling creature, a wraith. The Ancient Mariner, bearing the stigmata of another world, couldn't hold a candle to me back from Kerala. I sink into a chair and try to tell her my story. But my words are still muddled, I get things in the wrong order, or simply trail away. She looks appalled.

Two days later, thanks to the National Health Service, I have seen my GP, Dr Kaz (he has a much longer Polish name, but it's so full of 's's and 'z's that everyone calls him Kaz, and he doesn't mind). He's as perturbed as Jane at the way I look and move. I undergo a battery of tests, including an ECG, and am referred to the Hospital for Tropical Medicine in Gower Street, where a consultant goes over every scrap of my medical history. 'I think you may have a virus called Giardia, which can be caught in contaminated water,' he says, 'and even if you don't the antibiotics I'm going to prescribe will do you no harm.'

He makes an appointment a few days later for me to have an endoscopy and a colonoscopy – in which they slide a tiny camera down your throat and up your arse to check for any unusual growths. Time passes. I feel worse.

The night before the appointment, my stomach swells to late pregnancy size and I cannot sleep at all. Driving to University College Hospital with Jane next morning, wincing at the bump of every traffic sleeper, I mutter, 'They can't push a camera down me when I'm in this condition.' The surgeon at the Gastro-Enterology Department, Dr Karen Barclay, brisk and decisive, takes one look at my belly, shakes her head, and orders up an X-ray, rapidly followed by a CT scan when she sees there's something seriously wrong. She and her team examine the results, and she tells me I have 'a perforated colon' and need to have surgery. Urgently.

I drift in and out of sleep in my cubicle in the Admissions ward. It seems to be night-time when I wake and find Dr Barclay standing by my bed, looking tense. Keeping her voice down, she tells me that I have bowel cancer, and that if she doesn't operate soon, something even worse could happen to my stomach: the bowel could burst, depositing toxic matter everywhere. 'I hate operating at night,' whispers Dr Barclay. 'The back-up's not as good. But I warn you,' she adds, with an admonitory finger, 'if I detect the slightest sign of trouble, I'll go ahead anyway. We'll be monitoring you through the night.' There's a high-pressure tension about her; she reminds me of Electra approaching her decisive action. The static of electricity and danger hangs on after she sweeps out.

In the end, they do not operate overnight. Next morning the entire surgical team turn up to inspect me – Dr Barclay, her fellow consultant Dr Richard Cohen, and a gaggle of younger doctors. They mutter about 'Hartman's procedure'. I learn a week after the operation that this means removing the infected part of the colon, sewing up the rectum and punching a hole in the stomach, so the shit issues into a bag stuck to your skin. I now have a seam with stitches down my chest and a new aperture in my belly. Coming to terms with feeling that you're little more than a bag of shit which burps and grumbles does rather plant your feet firmly on the ground.

These incisions have been made to remove not just several inches of infected bowel but also a dozen lymphatic nodes – which have not been infected, a good sign, it seems. I am deposited, several ounces lighter, in the Intensive Care Unit, which may be higher in the tower of University College Hospital, or deep in its, I guess I have to say, bowels.

Once, a long time ago, returning on the sleeper train from Edinburgh after a night's serious drinking at the art school, I got out of bed in the cruel dawn, staggered to the mirror, and could have sworn I could see in the reflection my body still stretched out on the bunk. It was like that in Intensive Care. I felt distanced, dislocated; was this really happening to me?

Unfocused figures of nurses come and go in the hush of the Intensive Care Unit, where I wake in a refrigerated chamber. I manage a few sentences in my floating post-operative state. After two or three days, I'm able to see that Dr Karen Barclay is not only efficient but dashingly well-dressed – even her operating-theatre gown is stylishly cut. She reminds me of the attractive masterful women in J G Ballard's stories. Her colleague Dr Richard Cohen is an even snappier dresser. They tell me I have recovered enough to be moved to an ordinary ward. I tell them they are the best-dressed consultants in UCH.

I end up on the ninth floor, with rooftop vistas across London University and Bloomsbury as far as the London Eye can see. The ward is divided into four-bed cubicles. In the two beds facing me are Tom and Ivan. Tom is a flaxen-haired Glaswegian with a bewildered child's expression; Ivan, from Belfast, wears an ear-ring and a big black leather jacket with studs. They both lever themselves out of bed in the morning to go downstairs. 'To the café, like,' Ivan says; but I wonder whether it's a trip to the morning tipple. Later I find that Tom has cirrhosis. I never find out what Ivan has, because he discharges himself from the hospital a day later. As does their crony Richard, a beaky man who looks glum and ill. Tom tells me Richard is a well-read man, 'a scholar, knows all about the history of the First World War.' When he leaves, he doesn't look as if he has a home to go to.

If I was in a private clinic like the Wellington or the Cromwell, its big fees paid out of medical insurance, I'd never meet working-class men like Tom and Ivan, only rich people and foreign potentates. University College Hospital is a private/public enterprise; you can see it's not short of cash by the monumental size of the building, the quality of its interior finishes and its state-of-the-art technology. The big scanner comes from Germany, made by Siemens.

But the hospital doesn't feel like a commercial operation. I trust the consultants; the nurses, from Africa, the Caribbean, the Middle East and Eastern Europe, are quietly efficient. And humorous Karen Anderson, the senior nurse of my ward, is a tall, energetic Jamaican woman, always on the move, with a stream of music-hall repartee. She ribs Tom and Ivan as if they were naughty schoolboys, pitchforking them out when their beds have to be made, mock-sighing and raising her eyes to the skies when they resist her. She reminds me of Josephine Baker, the lanky American showgirl, who conquered Paris and became a French star. 'You should have been on the stage,' I tell her. 'I wanted to, but me mam couldn't afford the fees, so I was sent to nursing college,' she replies. She keeps the junior nurses on their toes, fills out clipboards, scurries from one needy patient to the next, escorts another to the hospice to die. She flirts with me in a non-serious way, and calls me 'Professor' because I'm reading a thick book.

Day by day, my circle of awareness and movement expands. With my drip-feed as a companion I get out of bed and walk, past the neighbouring cubicles, past the 'Beverage Booth' and the pay-television slot machines and drink dispensers. At the end of every corridor, a new vista of Bloomsbury is revealed to the view, a sight that is a tonic in itself, though it seems to be raining for most of my stay.

The doctors' team makes its rounds in the morning. Richard Cohen declares I'm making good progress, but then I have a secondary infection, and spend the night throwing up. Karen Barclay, visiting next day, says I need my stomach syringed, and does the unpleasant job herself. Who would have thought I had so much liquid in me? Weak as a kitten, I get by, and the following day I am warily back to my best, whatever that means in these circumstances.

My brother phones and comes in, bringing a bunch of DVDs – a boxed set of Woody Allen, Godard's *Breathless*, Louis Malle's *Lift to the Scaffold*, with Jeanne Moreau and a jazz score by Miles Davis. But I can't get my laptop to play them. I hoist myself up to the keyboard, and begin this chronicle of my days and nights. Often awake before dawn, I pee into a bottle and start typing. It's a lifeline.

My sister's in New York, anxiously phoning for news. Jane comes in every day. I gaze at her, more lovingly than ever, and see the strain on her face. She says I'm coping well, with humour and calm. Peter Brook rings from Paris, then from London; he's brought *Sizwe Bansi*

Is Dead to the Barbican. Friends come in with fruit, chocolate and books, layers of my life renewed by their presence, their worried faces and voices. I had not thought I had so many threads linking me to loves and friends. I've given too little care to this.

With Jane, I set up an e-mail distribution list, and she sends out contained bulletins about my state to friends around the world, and comes back with news of their replies. This e-mailing reduces the number of calls she gets inquiring after me, but still the burden of being my carer and the first port of call shows around her tired eyes.

One day I gingerly walk down the street with her on shaky legs, heading for Gordon Square. The lushness of its lawns staggers me, after my eye-diet of plastic surfaces and waste disposal bags. Teachers and students from London University picnic on the grass, framed in flower-beds. We sit outside the coffee kiosk, a couple resting in a London park. I return to the square alone in the following days, gaze and dream about Bloomsbury lives, then walk back along Tottenham Court Road, its digital electronic bazaars flaunting SONY, SHARP, JVC, PANASONIC; and selling stationery, Paperchase selling storage boxes and Muji youth clothes in muted colours; sofas made in Scandinavia, ethnically-styled tables and chairs from India. Bastions of Britishness – Sainsbury's, Heals – stand out from the globalised *soukh*, at least until they're taken over and franchised by foreign owners. Britishness as a brand. I know how much of it is born of the labour of low-paid Third World workers, but I still like the place, the stir of a market, the buzz of a world site.

Back in the ward, there's a new arrival in the bed between me and the window. Nachman is a copybook Orthodox Jew from Stamford Hill, a bony man not yet sixty but looking much older with his sallow skin and long beard, his little white *kippa* (the skull-cap Orthodox Jews perch on their head), his priestly robes, *tallith* and *tefillin*. He's flanked by two sons and a flock of relatives, friends and fellow-congregants, which soon grows to a flood. They take charge of their corner of the ward – and beyond. Goods and property are heaped everywhere. Hat-boxes – drum-shaped, made to carry Hasidic fur hats, one for weekdays and a special one for *Shabbos*, are planted on the window-sill, intruding on the view of the Bloomsbury rooftops.

In Hebrew, I introduce myself: '*Ani Yehudi,*' I am a Jew. They look at me blankly – Hebrew is for prayers, Yiddish is for talking, They didn't expect to find another Jew in this secular temple of healing in an alien land.

Nachman is sat up in bed, upright and supported by pillows, leaning forward over his bed-table, on which is placed a lectern to hold his small library of Hebrew prayerbooks. Nachman begins to *doven*, tracing the letters on the page with a long skinny finger, articulating the words for the umpteenth time in a rapid, scarcely audible mutter. Younger male relatives join him, and soon there's a little Orthodox congregation rocking and murmuring behind the closed cubicle curtains. Daylight fades, Nachman doesn't stop praying. Night falls and his flock departs, except for one of his sons, a big fleshy man who towers and fusses over his father.

Nachman goes on *dovening* into the night. I know this because the light from his cubicle spills into mine and keeps me awake until midnight. Tossing and turning, I catch glimpses of Nachman bent over his lectern, and behind him his son, who has told the nurses he's going to sleep all night in a chair by his father, completely breaking the rule that requires visitors to leave by 10pm. The nurses decide to let him stay. Later I catch another glimpse of Nachman through a gap in the curtain. Now he has fallen asleep, his head resting on his lectern, still, timeless, prayed out.

I'm struck by the total world these *frummers* (Orthodox Jews in Yiddish) bring with them, a kind of parallel universe that only rarely touches or communicates with the secular world around them. They have their own vernacular, their own dress code – black, invented in eighteenth-century Poland and worn ever since, whatever the climate. They 'marry in' – one of Nachman's many daughters is getting married in a couple of days' time, and he will get up for the wedding, no matter how sick he's feeling. At the ceremony and the celebration, the sexes will be divided; men will dance with men, women with women, a long curtain will divide male from female. The lust of the eye, the appreciation of the body, must be curbed.

Next morning, Nachman and I are awake early. He beckons me to come into his space, questions me about my life, my Jewishness, my wife. 'Partner,' I say, and tell him she's not Jewish. I imagine him thinking, 'Another Jewish boy lost to the tribe', but his face is a mask of soulful resignation.

That afternoon, Nachman introduces me to his future son-in-law, a sharp-featured, fast-talking young man. He and the other men in the cubicle are 'laying *tefillin*' – strapping leather thongs around their arm and head, each carrying a box with a scrap of parchment with a holy text. He asks me to join them. I haven't laid *tefillin* since my *barmitzvah*, fifty-five years ago. I'm tempted to join them, and besides it would be churlish to refuse their invitation. My father, could he see me now, might be proud of me, so I say yes, and follow the son-in-law's murmured instructions as I wrap the parchment texts close to my forehead and my heart.

Nachman smiles when we have finished, as if I've 'crossed over' to their world, albeit momentarily. He takes off his *kippa* and offers it to me. 'No, no,' I say. 'Take it, Michael,' he says, 'it means more to you than it does to me.' I wear it, feeling oriental. Next day, he looks painfully at it, and it's clear he'd like it back, so I give it to him. 'It's the special one I wear on *Shabbos*,' he says apologetically.

The sun is beginning to set as I make my way back to bed. The world of the *frummers* is hidden behind the curtain; I'm alone. But not for long. A dapper fifty-ish man appears from the direction of Nachman's bed. He's wearing the regulation long black coat, only his seems sharper and smarter, more tailored and of better cloth.

'My name's Avital. Avi,' he says. 'Where are you from?'

'Golders Green,' I say.

'You married to a Jewish girl?' he says.

I want to say, what business is it of yours, but instead I say, 'I was. Twice. But it didn't work out. I don't have children and I live with Jane, who isn't Jewish.'

'What made you choose a Jewish wife to start with?' he asks. He's as pushy with his questions as a detective, and seems impatient to get the information as fast as possible, and then move on. He doesn't pay much attention to my replies; his eyes shift restlessly over my shoulder, in search of more interesting prey. This is annoying.

'If you want to come in here and talk to me,' I say, 'you'd better pay attention. You can't just sit there and watch other people going by.'

I pull the curtains to, so he can't see. I find out that he's a property developer, but his real vocation seems to be visiting hospitals. This is his third hospital visit today and he will do two more, he tells me, before he goes home. He reels out their names – the Royal Free, Saint Mary's, the Marsden.

Trying to change the subject, I ask him if he's ever been to Israel.

'Never.'

'Aren't you interested to see what life is like there?'

'Not at all. We're happy to lead a hundred per cent Jewish life in Stamford Hill.'

'Don't you want to see Jerusalem?'

'No. Israel is an obstacle. Its existence delays the coming of the Messiah.'

'What made you marry Jewish girls?' he asks again. 'What's Jewish in you?'

I stumble trying to explain to my impatient listener. I talk about being a non-observant, 'non-Jewish Jew,' in Isaac Deutscher's phrase, about being a Jew culturally, but not in practice. Certainly not the kind of practice these Stamford Hill Jews observe, wrapping every hour of the day in prayers, obeying every observance codified in the Talmud. There's something moving about this communal identity – there would be if Avi were Muslim or Catholic – but there's also something repetitive and closed and stereotyped. The faithful have a tendency to become narrow and censorious. They demote women and revile homosexuals, ban books and excommunicate dissidents. Which is, I guess, why I got out of Golders Green. But how far have I travelled?

'Who are you under?' he suddenly asks.

Who am I under? What's he talking about? Oh, he means, which hospital consultants. I give him the names of my surgeon and my oncologist, both, as it happens, Jews. Avi smiles. 'I've known them since they were –' and he raises his hand to a *barmitzvah* boy's height.

'What do you do for a living?' he asks.

'I write.'

'Bestsellers?'

'Well no, not bestsellers. I just try to write well.'

Avi looks disappointed at my not being a bestselling author. He then reels out a long list of 'the best consultants' in the many London and Home Counties hospitals he visits. Getting tired of his name-dropping and his appointment-listing, of his incessant flow of words, I tell him he's well on the way to a heart attack, God forbid, if he doesn't slow down and take a break.

This brings him to a halt for a moment.

'But I can't stop. I mustn't stop. I have to find the best doctors if, God forbid, my family or my friends fall ill. Nachman, for example – I've been his friend and his counsellor for many many years. I got him a bed in this hospital. A couple of phone calls. He's going to die, you know. Cancer of the oesophagus. Incurable. But he won't tell his family. He needs me by his side.'

Is Avi what Christians would call 'a good Samaritan'? Is he what Jews would call a *mensch*, a decent man, or is he a *schwitzer*, someone who sweats with perpetual motion, busying himself to do good? Is he a busybody, filling his days with plans and activity, restlessly in motion, so he won't have to stop and reflect?

Later, when I'm out of the hospital, Avi rings me at home to see how I'm doing. He gets my surname wrong, and I realise he must have written it down on a piece of paper. I have become another target in the stream of Avital's attentions.

Coming Out

An agèd man is but a paltry thing,
A tattered coat upon a stick

I'm coming out
But will it go away?
I'm coming home
It travels with me

I'm standing up
It walks around
Up and down
My capillaries

I'm lying down
It starts to dance
Tom-tom feet
Along my gut

It hides its face
But has it gone?
It's taking cover
For how long?

It sits and grins
It has long teeth
It swells and spreads
And smiles like death

I am not it
It is not me
It occupies
My space and time

It pullulates
Through every cell
Carelessly choosing
To leave its mark

It's very fast
It never sleeps
Unwelcome lodger
In my flesh

When it made its appearance, I could not think about it. Its impact stunned thought. Later, on reflection…but reflection always comes later. What's it like? I cannot tell. I only know it's there, and know that I know.

I took cognisance of it very suddenly. An emergency. If they did not catch it, it would capture all my stomach. The urgency squads had to mobilise fast. They skipped scans in order to get to it fast. They knew enough to act. Tonight, if needs be. It was next day in the end. They hit the ground running; knocked me out fast; took it out as fast as they could make it.

I see a malevolent snake in a metal bowl. Slopmeat of sickness.

I am a passenger on your runaway train. You are the ticket collector; I have no ticket; you will throw me through the window off the train.

It hurts. I wake. It hurts. It won't let me sleep. Peppermint tea helped once, but no more. It kicks and shoves, a rude bedmate.

However it's treated, it never renounces its Right of Return. The harsher the treatment, the more fiercely it grips its Right.

'On reflection.'… Always later, too late. In the moment, nothing. I am Yeats' 'tattered coat upon a stick'; these lines my soul's singing.

'Soul'? A new tenant, never admitted to my word-room before.

It reminds me what a late starter I am. A late starter in the last chance saloon. Still time for a turn or two, though the front-cloth man may soon be snatched off by the cruel hook from the wings.

The feet tap-dancing, the mouth a rictus. The rectum blocked; use the bag provided for waste matter. It makes you feel lopsided? No matter; better than infection in the wound.

Learn to love your own shit. In Richard Hamilton's 1983 painting *The Citizen*, the prisoner, a republican, refuses to wear prison uniform. 'We are political prisoners,' said the prisoners. 'No toilets for anyone who doesn't wear the uniform,' replied the guards. The blanket prisoner in the painting paints his cell walls in his own shit: gestural marks like a Jackson Pollock painting, inside a Hamilton painting. Receding planes of reality. Turning a punishment into an opportunity.

I must be patient; scars take time to form. Time enough for me to get to know it, stop treating it as a stranger, change to meet it, make it mine, shape myself to the new worlds. Gulliver plunged into new worlds, first among the Thimble People, then the giants and then the Yahoos and the horses, powerless to protest, no time to linger on the first astonishment.

A dybbuk in my body. The surgeon my exorcist.

Keep alert. Heart failure, not just cancer, could get you in the end.

Monday, May 28, 2007

Discharged from hospital, I come home to my flat. Barry has painted all the walls a gleaming white. I decide to hang fewer pictures, let the white walls give me space. District nurses come to change the dressing on my wound. I'm settling back into my nest. I walk with care. Sunlight hits the garden, the apple trees, the squirrels, the mother fox and her lair. Friends turn up, sit and talk. I'm a lucky man.

Soon it's ten weeks since I set out for India. Now I'm living an aftermath, a passage from India.

Birds sing, sunshine bathes my head, I read, I fall asleep, I wake to read. Fernanda – more than my Portuguese cleaning lady, my friend – cooks me stews and soups and tell me how she's met Jose Mourinho. Jane takes stock. It's time she got out of the house, where my illness has trapped her. As soon as I'm able to look after myself, we plan to go to France, to stay with Adrian and Celia in an isolated house in the country. Then one day I realise I shouldn't go. If something were to go wrong with me, if I ran out of pills or needed a hospital, I'd become an unnecessary burden on everyone. I tell Celia that I'm not coming, and Jane that she should go anyway. I'll be all right in this garden, with friends and helping hands.

Friday, June 1, 2007

I write to the head of the clinic, the man who had impressed me with his noble bearing and quiet authority, Krishna Kumar:

Dear Krishna,

I wish I could tell you that the past few months have been happy ones. But the truth is that I arrived back in London after my stay on Coimbatore with fierce stomach pains, which I experienced from the time of my arrival at your clinic, and during my entire stay. In London before my departure, I thought it was some kind of stomach virus, but decided to come to your clinic rather than postpone my trip, because it was put to me that your doctors would be able to cure it there, as part of my overall treatment.

As my clinical notes will show, although different methods were tried, the stomach pain did not go away, and soon was preventing me from sleeping. The pain also began to affect my walking, so that I was shuffling and moving with difficulty. When I was discharged on March 10, I was not healthy. Indeed, it could be said that I should not have been discharged in the condition I was in.

I flew back to London via Sri Lanka on March 15. When I arrived at London's Heathrow airport, I was in bad shape. I managed to get home, where I was greeted by a horrified partner: I looked like a very sick man. I *was* a very sick man, and it may be said I am lucky still to be alive.

I was diagnosed as having cancer, with a perforated colon. The infected part of my bowel was removed at London's University College Hospital, and I will soon decide whether to start chemotherapy.

Krishna, I would much rather be writing to you about the good sides of my stay at Coimbatore, about the dedication of your staff and the Shakespeare workshop I so much enjoyed doing. I have not been well enough until now to tell you what has happened. But I am sorry to tell you that I do not believe I was given adequate care by the clinic's doctors, despite daily visits, and an examination by your chief medical officer. In your brochure for the clinic, you note that 'In the case of occurrence of any condition which our physicians think needs immediate attention, the Allopathic consultant will guide you and if necessary, we will make arrangements to take you to a nearby

Allopathic hospital which is well equipped to deal with such conditions.'

Krishna, despite the fact that I was in pain for my entire stay, it never occurred to anyone that I might need such a referral. All that was done was to adjust my diet, add some further medication and go easy on the massage when it came to my stomach. All with no effect. I do not regard this as responsible duty of care to a patient.

Krishna, the more I look at your brochure, the angrier it makes me. I read 'Just leave the decisions to the physicians and abide by what they say, and we assure you that everything we do will be only in your interest.' I did follow their instructions, while making it clear that my pain was not going away. The result is that I am lying in London as a cancer patient.

Maybe this would have happened anyway. But my point is that I was not given the benefit of due care that any responsible doctor owes to the patient. As it turned out in London, I received surgery only at the eleventh hour.

I wonder what you think of this treatment, Krishna – and also what my team of doctors thinks. I had good relations with them, but they clearly did not take me seriously when I said I had such bad pain in my belly that I could not sleep for night after night.

Perhaps it is my fault to some extent. I am not a complainer, and I was active within the clinic, offering you the Shakespeare evening for example, even when I was not feeling well (I left two days later). But the fact remains that I was discharged from the clinic in worse health than when I arrived.

I sign the letter 'in sorrow and in friendship'. There is no reply. I send it again. Eventually I get a reply from Krishna Kumar. It's brief, a sentence from a man with more pressing things to deal with. He says he will pray for me.

Chapter Five:
ÉMIGRÉ'S RETURN

July 2001

A suicide bombing was carried out by the Hamas member Hassan Khutari in a discotheque near the Dolphinarium in Tel Aviv, Israel on June 1, 2001 in which 21 Israelis were killed and more than 100 were injured.

In longshot, a bunch of people on the beach, somewhere between Tel Aviv and Jaffa. They look nomadic, out of place; they are not wearing beachwear, they're wearing Arab clothes. Close-up on one little girl talking to her family in Arabic on a mobile phone. 'We're on the beach, I'm seeing the sea for the first time.' Boys in the group scamper into the waves in jeans and T-shirts. Longshot: under a sun-shade, three middle-aged women in swimsuits are looking at the bunch of Palestinians. In Hebrew, one says sourly, 'They've come across to check out the place before they take it over.'

This is the opening of *The Inner Tour,* a feature-length documentary film which follows a group of Palestinians from the West Bank and Gaza on a three-day coach tour into Israel. Three days, because that's the duration of their entry permit. They visit places where they or their ancestors used to live until 1948, share memories of farms and businesses they used to have, compare stories of loss. They talk to Israelis: when the guide in a kibbutz museum displaying photographs of the Independence war tells them ten kibbutzniks were killed in 1948, they ask how many Arabs were killed. A man who has been in an Israeli jail asks a Tel Aviv taxi driver to take him to the place where Rabin was shot, because he met him when he visited the jail. He stands sadly by the Rabin memorial, with its pitifully few bunches of flowers.

They stare through the coach windows at irrigated fields and shiny tower blocks, such transformations, such wealth compared to the camps and towns where they now live. One says, 'We weren't good enough to deserve this country.' When they reach the garish Dizengoff shopping mall, one woman says, 'If people came here from the West Bank, they'd strip it like locusts.' You realise that these exiles live, not a continent away, but just an hour's bus ride from their previous life.

A commissioning editor friend at BBC Four called to ask if I could write about this film. He'd commissioned it from Israeli and Palestinian film-makers, who had shot it in Summer 2000, before the intifada made such collaborations impossible. He knew I was exercised by what was happening now between Israel and the Palestinians. But in Spring 2001 I couldn't place a piece about it in the British press. Maybe it was British pre-election fever, or Middle East compassion fatigue.

But I decided I want to show it to a Jewish, or mostly Jewish, audience, to trigger the kind of 'family' discussion among British Jews I'd been seeking. Since the disproportionate response of the Israeli army to the Jerusalem riots after Ariel Sharon's provocative Temple Mount walkabout in September 2001, I'd been aching for this debate.

The Inner Tour, directed by Ra'anan Alexanderowicz, an Israeli, and produced by Palestinians and Israelis, portrays without preaching the pain of exiled Palestinians, which most Diaspora Jews and Israelis have pushed away. As the attacks and retaliations in Israel and the Territories mounted, and calls came from outside to denounce and criticise, and from within myself to see more clearly and take some action, I'd been feeling like Macduff in exile.

As a member of Jewish Diaspora I felt that Jews needed to go on our own tour of the interior, so that our stance and actions might be based on acknowledgement and not dogma or denial. Showing *The Inner Tour* to a small sample of Jews in London in July 2001 would at least allow some of us to admit the sadness of ordinary Palestinians into our minds.

You get to know two Palestinian mothers in this film. The older one, Siham El-Ouk, comes from Aida refugee camp. She looks about 50, and you first see her shouting at her two boys to come out of the sea when she tells them. Her husband was killed in 1982, when Israel invaded Lebanon, and she's turned herself into an iron woman, a Hecuba steeling her sons for a harsh world. The younger mother, Jihad Salah from Bethlehem, whose husband is in jail for life for killing an Israeli soldier, is upset by the other's ferocity to her kids: 'When they grow up, they'll say: You gave us everything, except our childhood.'

In a fairground in Tel Aviv, while their children are enjoying dodgem cars, a labyrinth of mirrors and a shooting range (unsettling to see a Palestinian teenager carefully aiming a rifle at a target), Jihad Salah asks the older mother, 'What would you do if you met the Israeli who killed your husband?' 'If there was no chance of being found out,' replies Siham El-Ouk, 'I would tear him limb from limb.'

Jihad stares at her, stunned at her vehemence. Then she says, 'You know, the wife of the soldier my husband killed must feel like that.'

The screening, in a lecture room at the London School of Economics, is packed with 150 people. They've been invited through the internet, personal contacts that make the event something like the gathering of relatives I've wanted.

'I wanted to provide a forum for face-to-face talk to happen,' I say, 'like a discussion in a troubled family gathering. This film is not about the images of violence that fill our television screens. In a way, it's not about now; it's about how the lives of yesterday live on now. Something we Jews understand very well.'

I'm interrupted from the audience: 'Why do you say "we Jews"? There are people in the room who aren't Jewish.' I repeat that everyone's welcome, but I surely have the right to speak to the Jews in the room as 'we'. I hadn't realised what a minefield of nerve-ends I was entering.

A rough and tumble debate follows. The head of a philanthropic fund who has just returned from Israel thinks this is a bad moment to show this film, when Israelis are scared about their own survival. Someone else retorts that there will never be a good moment. A veteran of political meetings launches into a denunciation of the Zionist state. I ask him to stick with his personal response to the film, since we all know the arguments, but we've just shared an experience, a new recognition for some of us.

A young Palestinian woman says how grateful she is for this screening, and then cries out, 'You know what you have been doing to us! You are sophisticated people! How could you go on doing it!' And she subsides into tears. Most people are speaking from previous agendas, few are talking about what they've just seen, which is not an atrocity or propaganda film, but a patient picture of Palestinians in exile, just as Jews have been. Avi Shlaim, who in his books has cleared away much mythology from the history of the Israelis and the Arabs, likes the film 'because it humanises the Palestinians'. I want to ask, how did they get dehumanised? Can't we learn from what was done to us? Or must we be condemned to enact the violence of the former victim?

The day after the first screening, I e-mail the audience:

'Perhaps the most important thing is to find a way to enable individual Jews to "stand up and be counted" and to "bear witness" to the loss that has been inflicted on the Palestinians. A way that will overcome the objection "You don't live in Israel, so you have no right to speak".'

Then I am knocked sideways by an epic e-mail from my friend Joshua Sobol, the author of *Ghetto*. It's like a cry from a maddened Daniel in the lion's den.

Dear Michael

You write of 'the loss that has been inflicted on the Palestinians'.

By whom?

By their leaders who pushed them to assassinate Yosef Haim Brenner in 1921?

By their leaders who pushed them to start the killings of Jews in 1929, and the killings of Jews and Arabs in 1936, which ended up with the assassination of many Palestinian intellectuals by the frustrated and defeated Palestinian bandits and gangs?

The loss that has been inflicted on the Palestinians by whom?

By their leaders who rejected the UN decision on the partition of Palestine and opened war on the Yishuv in 1948?

By their leaders who unleashed some ten months ago the present wave of violence, thus smashing to pieces the fragile Oslo agreement, which postulated an end to the use of violence in any future case of contention?

The loss that has been inflicted on the Palestinians by whom?

By that cynical liar Arafat, who has managed to smash to pieces the Israeli Left, which was the only political force in the world that could help his poor Palestinian people get a state of their own? Or do you believe that any individual Jew or group of Jews in the world is capable of helping him to climb out from the murky mine of shit into which he plunged the Palestinians with his treacherous, terrorist activities? Or do you still believe that any nation or group of nations besides Israel will be able to offer the Palestinians an independent state?

The greatest irony of the history of Israel and the Palestinians is the fact that it was only the Israeli Left that really cared about the Palestinians, and it is that slandered and besmirched Israeli Left that lifted Arafat to his feet, restored the plucked feathers from his crown, and brought him over to Palestine from his sweet *galut* in Tunisia, made him a persona grata in the White House, offered him an honest agreement, fought to change public opinion in Israel, and managed to create a majority in Israel for a peace agreement with the Palestinians.

And it was Arafat, that pathological liar, who, like the scorpion in the fable, stung the frog that was carrying him over the water; and, like the scorpion in the fable, carried out his stupid, suicidal crime before reaching the shore, and now he is yelling and crying for help, because he is drowning.

So let me tell you this: let this stupid scorpion drown. This is the only thing that he has earned honestly.

But if you wish to play the part of a new frog – please, jump into the water, swim to him and invite that drowning scorpion to get on your back. You will certainly earn his words of flattery while he is riding on your back, as we did, we the Israeli Left, before he will sting you, as he did us. And when you ask him why he did it, he will reply that it was all your fault, because you believed that he could overcome his scorpion's nature.

To be serious for a change, I believe that any activity, of individual Jews or grouped leftists or marginal vegetarians, in support of the present Palestinian Authority is in the long run working only against the Palestinians, and in favour of the Israeli Right. It may seem paradoxical to you, but there is nothing that the Israeli right wing is praying for now as much as conscience-cleaning activities on the part of Jews and Leftists, because this is the best and historically proven recipe to boost Palestinian Illusionism. It was Palestinian Illusionism that brought upon that miserable tribe the calamity of 1948, and Palestinian Illusionism that drove them to reject Barak's and Clinton's offers. All the Palestinians need these days is another boosting of their innate or acquired Illusionism to lead them to a frontal clash with Israel.

Afterwards you will be able to speak once more of 'the loss that has been inflicted on the Palestinians' and you may also wonder by whom it was inflicted.

Forgive me my uncontrolled outburst, but I am sick and tired of the abuse of goodwill and the abuse of language in the case of the rotten Israeli/Palestinian conflict. I think that if there is any chance to find some way out of it, it consists in the first place in abandoning the redundant vocabulary that accompanied us during the last three decades – or rather, ever since this conflict started, some hundred years ago, and some say even earlier.

I returned last week from a fortnight in Lithuania, where I have been working with a young Lithuanian film director on the second draft of a script for a film based on my play *Ghetto*, which will be shot in Vilnius, on authentic locations. One weekend we went to the Baltic resort of Nida, not far away from Kaliningrad, which had been Koenigsberg once upon a war. I was told that in 1944, when the Russians occupied that beautiful town, they kicked out all its German inhabitants overnight. They were sent away to share the fate of another seven or eight million Germans forced to leave their homes and villages and towns in what had been eastern Prussia.

Does anyone, except for neo-Nazis, bring up the question of 'the right of return' of those millions of Germans who had to suffer the consequences of belonging to a nation that started a war and lost it? Does anyone deplore 'the loss that has been inflicted on the poor Germans,' or do we all agree that that loss was inflicted upon them by their criminal leaders? Do you not think that Amin El Husseini, who was the Mufti of Jerusalem, and an ally of Hitler, should be held responsible for the historical loss that he has inflicted upon his people? Why Hitler and not Amin? Thank you for your response to my letter. I simply couldn't control my fingers running on the keyboard. The situation here is quite alarming, with winds of war gathering around us. Can we still do anything to stop this useless war from breaking out? Does it still depend on us at all? One more Dolphinarium incident with a score of victims, and a full-scale onslaught on the Territories will become inevitable.

I am looking forward to reading your enlarged response.

Dear Joshua

I regret that my e-mail about 'the losses inflicted on the Palestinians' made you lose an afternoon of writing. But maybe your eruption is part of *The Tragedy of Israel*, the play you are writing, and which I long to see. Because I love your plays, and respect you as a playwright of Jewish history and dilemmas, a European author and a toucher of moral nerve ends. Your letter overflows with personal passion, and yet has the dramatist's 360 degree impersonality, the ability to stand outside oneself. Well, to some extent. Your first reaction was to call me naïve. There have been others like it from Israeli friends who are angry with what they think is my 'position'.

But the truth seems different to me. Yeats said that 'the best lack all conviction, while the worst are full of passionate intensity'. Even those who hold similar convictions – and I sense that yours and mine, as Jews of the Left, are not far apart, even if we are geographically distant – are set against each other by 'the sins of the fathers'.

A psychotherapist friend, who could not help hearing me shouting down the telephone during a family quarrel, said, 'When there is trauma in the family, the parents set the siblings against each other.' There's been no lack of trauma in our generic Jewish family, and maybe my indignation and your rage are symptoms of the siblings in question. Welcome to the Semitic family roadshow, a gladiatorial contest which will run and run and run, as the world looks on from the roadside and gives a thumbs up or a thumbs down for who shall live or die. Will it ever end?

You tell me that the play you are writing is called *The Tragedy of Israel*. There certainly is a tragedy, even if the world may have lost the faculty of responding to or even recognising tragedy. You could argue, as Avi Shlaim documents in *The Iron Wall*, that Israel's leaders have missed almost as many opportunities to begin peace as the Palestinians. Tragedy, however, does not arise from a competition as to who makes the greatest number of errors. Tragedy comes from blindness. Oedipus was blind long before he put out his eyes. Antigone is blind to everything except the righteousness of her cause; so is Creon. She sacrifices her life; he loses his son.

The blindness that has been so tragic in the making of a Jewish state came home to me again when my friend Michael Zander, an eminent emeritus law professor, gave me a pamphlet written by his father. Walter Zander fled Germany for Britain in the 1930s, became Secretary of the British Friends of the Hebrew University, and wrote *Is This The Way?: A Call to Jews* in 1947. It contains these uncomfortable words: 'If we search through all that we have said and written through all these years to prove our case, we shall find that we have said everything to stress our need, but that we omitted one thing which might have changed the whole relationship with the Arab. Never in the thirty years' argument have we admitted that our return, justified as it appears to us, inevitably requires from the Arab a sacrifice of the first magnitude – the sacrifice of giving up his right to rule himself.'

Over half a century later, after all the 'illusionism' (not confined to the Arabs) and hubris, the violence and counter-violence, these words speak about a blindness which remains tragic. We could not see, did not want to see, the children of Shem who are our brothers and sisters. And the media-fed mythologies, the melodramas of defeat and compensation on which most nationalism is built (look at the Serbs), the Bible-thumping, blinkered and resentful fundamentalism, the geo-political manoeuvres making Israel a 'front-line state' in the Cold War, have not benefited anyone's vision.

When this documentary film *The Inner Tour* came along, I knew I needed to gather a bunch of Jews to experience an outstanding documentary film together, to argue and to act, whatever action means in the current circumstances. I wanted to get to the brink of a civil war of words between Jews. I wanted it as a Jew and a British citizen, who nearly settled in Israel in 1961, has been married to an Israeli, has family and friends there. For in what looks like a lurch towards another war in the Middle East, I believe that British Jews, and Diaspora Jews, as a whole, should not give automatic adherence to threatened Israel, should not otherwise keep their mouths shut.

I know how enraged you feel about Arafat and the damage to the Israeli Left, but isn't he the only game in town, as Uri Avnery says? Last night BBC television continued its series about the tortuous progress towards a peace agreement in Ireland. Gerry Adams, leader of Sinn Féin, the political wing of the IRA, was certainly reviled by many as the hated Arafat figure of the conflict. And yet, as you know, such ambiguous, transitory figures often hold the baton in the relay-race of history. And on it goes.

You and I do not lack conviction, we're not made to live pragmatically. We inhabit different places, and our histories overlap but do not coincide. What is certain is that we are both surrounded by loud ignorance, sentimental myth, primitive fundamentalism, and fear which explains much but does not justify stupidity and the violence of former victims.

Dear Michael

I agree with you that the most fatal error one can commit in our situation consists in sticking to convictions. If I gave an impression of indulging in that sin, I want to make it clear beyond any doubt that the last eight months of violence left me stripped of any convictions whatsoever regarding our predicament.

If we find time and leisure for a more philosophical dialogue, I could enlarge on my present feeling of a gaping void wherever I had any convictions at all in the past. Now to the Ghetto film project. I am trying to get some Israeli producer interested in co-operating with the project. I feel it will be a shame if this film, dealing with such a Jewish subject, will be finally done as a co-production of Lithuanians, Dutch and Germans without any Jewish involvement or meaningful contribution to the production, except for the screenplay that I have written, and I am, after all, still Jewish, whatever that means.

My best to you, Joshua

On screen, *The Inner Tour* keeps throwing up understated but heart-wrenching images of exile and attachment to the land. We first see Wa'el El-Ashqar in the tour bus. He comes, the caption tells us, from Ramallah. He appears to be talking to his own lap. It turns out he's recording a message into his camcorder, its lens turned up to his face.

'I can't tell you how much I miss you, and worry that you're all right,' he signs off one message.

We don't know who he's making his videotape for until much later in the film, when, away from the group, he approaches a tall wire fence. Through its mesh, we see the distant figure of a woman, waving madly and screeching his name across the barrier. Then we realise that it's the border between Lebanon and Israel, that as a Palestinian he is not allowed in, and that these howls across 200 frontier metres are the closest he can get to his mother. He takes out the videotape and hurls it over the fence to her, and they part, waving, her voice a bird-screech of misery. In the next shot he is sitting by the roadside, slumped in immobile sadness.

Dear Michael

I have received Ra'anan Alexandrowicz's *The Inner Tour*. It is a very strong and sad document. It does leave you with a feeling of empathy with the suffering of the Palestinians and with their loss. I am showing it to friends, and all react in a similar way.

I am working on the second draft of my so-called *Israeli Tragedy*, and will get an English version ready as soon as I can.

Today we are having a meeting between Israeli Arabs and Jews in the Arab village of Kalansuwa, not far from Tul Karem. It all started with a meeting of eight people in Tel Aviv a month ago. We were a forum of six Jewish Israeli writers and university professors, and two Israeli Arab professors preparing a large public meeting in Nazareth to work out a new covenant between Israeli Arabs and Jews. I will tell you more about it when we return from Kalansuwa. Joshua.

In *The Inner Tour*, Abu Muhammed Yehia is the oldest man in the bus. He must be in his seventies, and the only one wearing traditional robes and head-scarf. He comes from Jelazun refugee camp. His face is wrinkled, burnished, crone-like. He squats with his walking stick in the kibbutz museum as the guide tells the official story. His bright blue eyes sweep the space. Otherwise he is utterly immobile.

After the group visits a little mosque in Acre, he halts outside. They gather round him, for he is an elder and a Haji, he has made the pilgrimage to Mecca, and his impromptu sermon in this mosque garden under the stars must be listened to.

'Dear brothers,' cries this old man, summoning all his energy, for he may never see this place again:

> Our hope comes from seeing how lovely the land is. And our pain from opening the wounds and the memories. As you know, brothers, all nations have holidays. East and West of us, from Rome to Circassia, they celebrate their feasts and sing their songs. And for us, every day is a wedding day for convoys of the dead, marching on the other side of the river. And those funerals never stop following us. Years and days pass, but for us, time stands still. How long will it be this way? I cannot say. But patience and faith have been our way. We stand steadfast, our feet embedded in our land. And from here, by the al-Jazzar mosque in Acre, we say: 'Let no one doubt. We are a people that won't disappear, and won't die. We will have our celebration. With God's help, it will come soon.'

It's hard as a Jew to watch this, to hear the old man's voice lifted in affirmation, and not recall *L'shana Ha'baa Yerushalayim*, 'Next year in Jerusalem', spoken by the same kind of old men, in the same kind of voice, through centuries and continents of Jewish exile.

At the end of the film, Abu Muhammed Yehia signals to the driver to stop the bus. He hobbles down and sets off scampering through the fields as best he may, clearing a path through long grass with his stick, slashing at the grass until he finds the herb he's looking for. He tears at its leaves, stuffs one in his mouth, chews and savours the remembered taste. Then he's off again, stumbling through the leaves, until he arrives at an unremarkable corner of a now foreign field, kneels to pray, and, as a mother and child arrive anxiously after him, turns to them and says, 'This is my father's grave.' And then, handing the child a bunch of his herbs, 'Eat it. It's delicious. But take care of the thorns.'

Dear Michael

I am writing these words a few hours after the latest massacre that took place this afternoon in the heart of Jerusalem, and after having watched the mob on the streets of Beirut and Ramallah rejoicing and celebrating that bloodbath, howling and hopping and bouncing and waving their limbs in all directions in a wild explosion of *Schadenfreude*.

I am afraid the rich English language is short of the precise equivalent for that German term describing the lowest degree of moral depravity: rejoicing at the disaster of another human being. I saw two religious leaders, one from Islamic Jihad and the other from Hamas, expressing joy and satisfaction at the slaughter of civilians, most of them women and children. One of those leaders was standing on the roof of a central building in Gaza, whipping up the mob to an orgiastic ecstasy.

When I saw that sordid show, I said to myself: here are the most hideous war criminals who are committing one of the basest crimes against humanity in front of the entire world. Here are so-called religious leaders who are poisoning the heart and soul of their own people with lethal hatred. Here they are in the act of preparing the next catastrophe for their own people. Observe them *in flagrante*, and remember them when the time comes to ask who carries the responsibility for the loss inflicted upon the poor Palestinian people.

I tried to imagine those religious leaders on the roofs of Gaza and Beirut, exhorting the crowd instead to remember that 'When your enemy falls, do not rejoice, and when he is defeated let not your heart frolic, lest God see it and find it evil'. But those religious leaders are obviously godless, and as far from the human wisdom and moral level expressed so succinctly in that phrase of Proverbs 24:17 as the sun is from the heart of darkness.

I look at those leaders, and I pray for their miserable people whom they lead to perdition.

But if the Book of Proverbs with its profound ethical and practical wisdom does not figure in their breviary, it is part and parcel of our scriptures and to my mind it expresses the quintessence of what practical Judaism should and could strive to become. And when I turn the page of my Bible to read the next chapter of Proverbs, I find another pearl of practical wisdom. It is Proverbs 25:21, which recommends that 'If your enemy is hungry, feed him bread, and if he is thirsty give him water to drink'. If you think this smells of Christian over-righteousness or of Kantian heroic ethics, the author of Proverbs hastens to explain that by feeding your starving enemy with bread and water, you 'pour out glowing embers on his head', and God will reward you for this. This doesn't mean that you set your enemy's head on fire, but that by doing this you reduce his hatred to ashes, and God will recompense you by transforming your enemy into your friend.

The ethics and the wisdom contained in that one phrase of Proverbs should strike an echo and resound in the mind and heart of every Israeli who grew up with the Hebrew of the Bible as the basic music of life. And here is one of the questions that makes my sleep wander in the heat of the nights of our blazing Israeli Summer of 2001: are we sensitive enough to the hunger and thirst and suffering of the people who hate us in the blockaded Palestinian villages and towns of Gaza and of the West Bank?

Another question torments me and makes my sleep wander in that endless night after the massacre perpetrated by Hamas in Jerusalem 12 hours ago. It has to do with the contagious power of hatred. When you see those masses celebrating the mass-murder committed by their *shahid*, their blessed martyrs, and dancing on the blood of the victims, you feel how easy it is to be filled with fury against that human aberration, how easy to hate those people who dance in the streets of their towns, and you catch yourself saying: 'God, they remind me of those other masses who screamed and shouted and yelled their hatred in the streets of Munich and Nuremberg'. Listen carefully to the voices of their leaders: are they preparing the hearts of their hordes to a genocide? If that is the case, we shouldn't allow ourselves to make the slightest mistake.

I know one thing for sure: no Israeli ever went to war with joy in his heart. Remember what happened in this country 20 years ago, when Begin and Sharon started a war that wasn't imposed on us. The consensus was torn to pieces. While the fighting was still raging in Lebanon, the streets of Tel Aviv saw one huge anti-war demonstration after another, and finally it was that stubborn Israeli anti-war civil revolt, and not the Hizbollah, that forced our government to pull our army out of Lebanon.

This is not the case with those acts of terrorism perpetrated in the heart of our towns. These acts give off a very bad smell of mass-murder – I would even dare to coin the term 'mini-genocide'. Don't you see that the 'limited' number of victims is due only to the physical limits of the size of a bomb that a suicide-terrorist can carry on his body without being too visible in a crowd of innocent people? Those leaders who call each of their people to kill his personal Jew, would they hesitate to equip their *shahids* with micro-nuclear-bombs if such mass-destructive devices were at their disposal?

I put that question because people who dance on the blood of children are genocidal. If that is so, what should we do? Let me push the question one step further: If that is so, what should you do? What should the European Community do?

The bomb that went off yesterday in Jerusalem, like the one that exploded in the Dolphinarium a few weeks ago, is not just one more act of blind terrorism. No. The word GENOCIDE is written in big letters on those acts. Can't you read it?

Dear Joshua

'Why, this is hell, nor am I out of it.' Christopher Marlowe's Faustus had a hotline to where we are. Isn't that where we are now: hell here on earth, the heart of darkness, as you say: the lynch mob exultant, the bonds of humanity snapped, joy in another's torment?

Last week, a bomb went off among the bars and food joints of Ealing, in West London. It was claimed by the 'Real IRA,' and was an eleventh-hour attempt to dish the peace process. Though it didn't kill anyone, there could well have been *Schadenfreude* among the perpetrators if it had. But no one would claim that they had been preparing the genocide of the British. Britain is not at risk, as Israel may be, and none of us outside can gainsay your alarm.

We face the extreme republican 'Real IRA' and the Protestant 'Red Hand' faction; you face Hamas and Islamic Jihad; the Palestinians face Kahane-ists and settler vigilantes who froth hate-speech just as much as your crowd-goading clerics.

There's a void because of the absence of leaders, on either side, who can pull their peoples back from the brink, maybe the nuclear brink, from which there is no way back, and you can buy miniature nuclear devices in the post-communist black markets. Is there a Mandela in the house? The Middle East has a job vacancy.

Thursday, June 28, 2007

Another about-turn. A few days ago I began to wheeze and breathe with difficulty. By Sunday night, three days before I was due to start chemotherapy, I was awake after two hours' sleep, unable to take or expel more than the shallowest of breaths. I tried to stem the thing with my usual remedies: peppermint tea and sweet pastilles. Outside in the garden, where I went to breathe, the air was damp and clinging. Just the conditions, I thought, to trigger asthma. I turned on the desk-fan to full and pointed it at my face. It was easier to breathe, but I was trapped: beyond the fan's reach I was gasping for air again. I turned the fan round and sat in its stream on the settee to watch a DVD until sleep might creep up on me. Miklos Jancso's soldiers chased each other across the Hungarian countryside. There were firing squads, single men throwing themselves into the river to escape enemy cavalry, an obscure reckoning between early twentieth century forces – Magyars, White Russians, Cossacks. This blur of conscripts and partisans in a vast landscape recalled my recurring war dreams.

I shifted on the settee, decided to try to sleep on it, in the fan's benevolent cold stream. Hopeless: the moment I lay down, the grip on my throat and air tubes tightened. I resigned myself to spending the rest of night sitting up, foreseeing the weariness that would eat into my bones the following day. Then I said, don't be stupid, get yourself to a hospital. I called the out-of-hours National Health, a voice called back, took my symptoms. A tall, bony Greek-Cypriot doctor arrived, listened to my chest and lungs, ordered an ambulance and soon I was back at University College Hospital Accident and Emergency, a face-mask of oxygen keeping me going.

Two days later, still in the Acute Admissions Unit, eased by drugs to steady my heart-beat and get rid of the water in my ankles and lungs, I asked my oncologist if I was strong enough to take the chemotherapy I was due to begin later that day. 'Certainly not,' he said. 'This breathing episode shows that chemotherapy would raise your risk of heart failure from one in ten to one in seven. I'm not giving you chemotherapy today, and the way things are, you may never have it.'

'But if I don't do chemo, what is my treatment?'

'A check-up every six months and regular monitoring.'

'But the chemo was meant to put me out of reach of any recurring cancer.'

'The extent to which your chances of not having a cancer recurrence is outweighed by the threat of a blood clot and a stroke.'

So it's choose your exit door. A trade-off. My bruised heart, afflicted by atrial fibrillation – a weakness of the heart's upper chambers which affects blood circulation – is excused from the encounter with chemotherapy, and whatever side effects there might have been. 'Risk/benefit,' says the nurse when I tell her what's been decided. Decided for the time being, anyway: I am inured to the fact that doctors don't pin themselves down with precise prognoses or deadlines. When I'd asked how long I have to wear my colostomy bag, and empty out my own waste, one doctor said, 'Six months,' overlapping with another who said, 'At least a year.'

The result of this *volte-face* is a shift in my focus: I now see myself, and maybe I am labelled in the clipboards, as a heart case with cancer, rather than a cancer case with a heart condition. Who do I talk to first? Oncologist or cardiologist?

The sudden reversal is another unsettling example of the turning-point which in classical Greek theatre was called the *anagorisis*, the pivotal moment when the protagonist recognises the real opponent and realises he has been labouring under delusions, struggling against phantom enemies. Famously, Oedipus comes to realise that his true enemy and the cause of the plague that is afflicting Thebes, is himself.

It's dizzying, this turning on a sixpence. I need a break. I put on shoes and go out for a coffee. In Whitfield Street I find a Brazilian coffeeshop, and sit outside trying to take in this Pirandellian perspective shift, this overturning of my world, the scenery spun round to reveal a different landscape. Another lesson in the fragility of appearances.

When I get home, I describe my turn-arounds in e-mails to friends, and am touched, stirred at times amazed at the responses they evoke. People imagine I am still in hospital, a bed-ridden creature crushed by medical misfortune. Or is it that they take what I'm going through more seriously than I do? Some friends, getting news of my cancer for the first time, scramble to respond, feeling they must say something before it's too late. There are a surprising number who have already experienced cancer or have someone close to them who has it.

'I got a shock this morning when I opened your e-mail. I knew nothing about what's been happening to you. The last I knew you were in a clinic in India enduring Ayurvedic treatments. I'm presuming that you've just had an operation. And that the progress is good.'

'Adrian informs me that you are in hospital, but impossible to confine to your room and treating your hospital like Claridges.'

'Hang on! day by day, week by week, from one pleasure to another, from one productive chore to the next. That is how healthy people also should be living their lives. With an appreciation of the feast that life is good (despite everything) and with a sense of one's own mortality. The rest is sheer arrogance.

I have been living with diabetes for almost 25 years now and the illness has taught me some humility, made me appreciate my time (so not to waste it) and relish pleasures and exciting experiences when available. That also means investing myself in friendships.'

'The odd thing is that five weeks ago I was in Italy and Ann rang me to say that she'd just been diagnosed with a cancer. She's now half way through a course of radio therapy and enduring the first (of two) sessions of chemo. The prognosis is very encouraging. A 95 per cent chance of a complete recovery. All she can do is grit her teeth and get on with the treatment. "It never rains but it pours," as they say up north.'

'Your e-mail was the first I knew of your battle with cancer. Thank God – or whoever – that you have come through it and are now back home. I was shocked by your news but since you are a man of extraordinary resilience and determination, I am in no way surprised that you seem to have come through the worst stage.'

One friend refers to my 'setback', a word which I refute, telling her there are benefits as well as setbacks and losses in what has happened to me, what I have happened upon. Sometimes I feel like a Buddhist, or what I imagine Buddhist equanimity would be, seeing this surgical excision and emotional destabilisation as part of the flow of life. Talk about 'setbacks' seems…excessive, somehow.

Saturday, June 30, 2007

Quizzical. That's the word I seized on in hospital when I found myself out of step with groaning, complaining fellow patients. Nurses praised my sense of humour, but in truth I used humour as a device to lighten – I hope not a shield to deny – the load my body was putting on me. And more, it seemed right to be quizzical because, in this world of sudden new symptoms and rapidly revised diagnoses – what Grace Paley calls *Enormous Changes at the Last Minute* – every assertion was liable to be reversed from one day to the next. My transformation from primarily cancer patient to primarily heart patient was a case in point. I'm both, of course, but suddenly the latter definition seemed to pre-empt the former, to seize the foreground from it. Now, although I know my surgeons and my oncologist by name and by face, I can't remember seeing a cardiologist in the same way, and I'd like to know what my own over-accelerated ticker is going to let me do in five or ten years' time. Assuming I last that long.

On such shifting sands, who could be sure of anything? Seeing the paradoxes quizzically and the contradictions dialectically seems a better choice, and that means seeing round the edges of your complaint, speaking of it with some lightness. The fatal knock at life's door has not yet arrived, and may not do so for a long time; I can still afford to quiz my condition.

This doesn't mean I've succumbed to relativism. Jane tells me how much more open and listening I've become, aware of my fellow human beings, curious about their lives. It's true I've relished the unpredictable encounters which hospitals present, found myself more undefended and responsive, even more charitable. Maybe medical misfortune can produce human gain, charity. A loss that knocks you sideways can engender comedic awareness of the flimsiness of human states and conditions; perhaps this is the basis of the Jewish joke, product of oppression, rebellion against resignation. Taking things too literally, too solemnly, would be an error. Two actors meet on the street. One's carrying a cigar-case. 'Working?' asks the first. 'Moving,' replies the man with the cigar-case.

Other patients around me, dislocated by their new sense of vulnerability, took shelter in complaining. Or in their faith – reading holy scriptures and sacred texts, sheltering in the brotherhood of churches and sects. The Father from a Bloomsbury church across the ward, suffering from heart damage, was visited by a succession of young congregants and priests. They conversed parochially.

Downstairs there was 'The Chaplaincy', a non-denominational chapel for prayer and contemplation, which I passed on my way to the café. Euston Road traffic flowed past this oasis of calm. But I did not see anyone going into or coming out of its tidy interior.

As the sixtieth anniversary of India's independence approaches, I see London filled with retrieved memories and images. A scale model of the Taj Mahal – which Tagore called 'a teardrop on the cheek of time', and which has just been voted one of the new Seven Wonders of the World – floats past the Houses of Parliament on a barge, to launch London's 'New India Festival'. At the British Library there is an exhibition going up, with text and pictures – Gandhi, Nehru – telling modern India's story. Television, which has had a love affair with the British Raj since Paul Scott's *The Jewel in the Crown*, programmes a brace of documentaries which cater to collective nostalgia with old photographs and shaky film of imperial British grandees at march-pasts and polo matches. Their descendants recall servants and *ayahs* and hill stations beneath the Himalayas. There's just one film from the viewpoint of ordinary Indian people – *Bombay Dreams*, a portrait of the teeming commuters on the railways that stitch together the packed segments of India's fastest-growing city.

New Indian fiction – Vikram Seth, Pankaj Mishra, Kiran Desai – fills the paperback shelves of London's bookshops. The English National Opera stages *Satyagraha*, Philip Glass's opera about Gandhi and non-violence. Andrew Lloyd Webber puts on a musical, *Bombay Dreams*. Bollywood DVDs sell in Brick Lane and Southall like hot samosas. The Anglo-Indian romance continues.

I ransack my shelves for books about India I have bought but not read, discs I have neglected. A comparison of Eastern and Western religions, written in the nineteen-thirties. Sanskrit play-scripts.

Monographs on Moghul architecture. The rousing, infectious syncopated rhythms of *tabla* and *sitar*, spinning out of long, reflective
mourning *ragas*. Albums of illustrated *vedas*, videos of *The Mahabharata*, Peter Brook's nine-hour theatre version of it, which, even
more than the films of Satyajit Ray with which I grew up, planted
seeds of India-philia in me.

I try to pick my way through the Western projections onto India,
the romantic relish of its pungent colours, seductive vocal melismas,
tickling spices and maddening smells. I warily note the adventures
of ashram-seeking, guru-worshipping devotees and their Californian
swamis (Isherwood and Huxley both sat at their feet), remembering
a macrobiotic meal in the 'sixties with John Lennon and Yoko Ono
in which their exalted enthusiasm for all things Indian was punctuated by the sounds of our soft farting after a dish of beans and
other pulses. I go to the Victoria and Albert Museum and gaze at
the exquisite residues of maharajah courts and British imperial rule.

Before I left for India, I made sure I saw Jatinder Verma, director
of Britain's longest-lasting Asian theatre group, Tara Arts. With his
silky beard, delicate build and steady gaze, Jatinder reflects back an
India that calmly takes in its stride invasions, eruptions and enthusiasms that would have convulsed other nations, smaller not only in
their geography, but in their mental and, I have to use the well-worn
word at last, their spiritual dimensions.

July 2007

I've been thinking about London as a city of confluence.

Our laundry-man is called Amir and comes from Iran. This
morning, when he comes bearing crisp sheets and tablecloth wrapped
in clear plastic, I ask him if we can talk about Iran. We stand by the
front gate in the sun.

He tells me he left after 'the Revolution', when the mullahs took over from the Shah. He was working as an accountant in a big company. He didn't have a beard and he wasn't much in evidence at the mosque. He soon began to realise that, unlike his orthodox, observant colleagues, he was being held back at work: no promotion, no salary rise.

Then the war with Iraq broke out. The Iraqis bombed a power station near his house. His son, taking cover under a table, was terrified by the explosions. The war went from bad to worse for the Iranians, and soon young boys were being conscripted, given a rifle and sent out to the desert to die.

Amir did not want this fate for his son. He contacted a friend, another accountant, who had left for London, and asked him to send a letter of invitation, saying he needed Amir for his business. This helped Amir get a visa, despite the vast queues at the embassy.

In London, he and his wife and son lived in one room with an Indian landlady. In Teheran, he had had a four-bedroom bungalow, and now he was in one room in Willesden.

He worked on a construction site, and then started his laundry business.

He suddenly asks me if I work for the newspapers. No, I say, I just write books. I tell him I would love to visit Iran, see Isfahan, Shiraz.

Later this day, I am having coffee in the Algerian patisserie shop in Crouch End. Two young women are sitting at the next table, talking with excitement. One of them mentions Iran. I ask her if she thinks the great Iranian films that have flowed out over the past eight years will be able to continue being made. After all, Iran's prime minister Ahmadinejad has already banned American programmes and films from state television. It doesn't make any difference, she says, most people have satellite. And anyway, Ahmadinejad realises that 60 per cent of the people are twenty or under, so he has to keep them happy to stay in power. He will balance between hard-line Islam and 'opium injections of things young people like'.

I like that phrase, I tell her. When Marx used opium as a metaphor, it was in reference to religion. Now secularism is the new opium of the people.

Later, in search of a good print shop in Soho, the hub of London's cosmopolitanism, I am directed to a basement Internet café in St Anne's Court. A young man brings a scanner and talks while his fingers guide my pages through the process. He is Russian, Alex is his name. His father, he says, is 'head of the CID in Moscow'. He's not keen to go back, doesn't want to be sent to Chechnya to fight. Confluence city, metropolis of meetings.

I go to Selsey, Sussex for ten days' R & R *chez* Pamela Howard.

Pamela's house is bursting with stories. The stories of the plays she has designed, the stages she has made – a traverse in a cavernous hall in Edinburgh, an open-air auditorium in a Venetian fortress in Thessaloniki. More stories on the Czech and Polish tea-towels with which she has hung her walls – embroidered comic strips of a woman in the kitchen cooking, shopping, sweeping. A feminist friend told her she was betraying women by displaying this woman doing all the unpaid labour, though to tell the truth the woman looks as if she resents cooking as little as Pamela, an inspired and improvisatory cook. More stories: the faces and figures on posters of her theatre work and the paintings and sinuous drawings she has done of characters in her plays and of people observed during rehearsal. Drawings like whispers. The story above all of her love affair with red and green: her house is a riot of blossoms, her garden a sea of vivid flowers. Sweetpeas erupt from jugs in a dazzle of purple and red, the cushions are orange and red, the chairs – some of them props from the nursery scene in *The Cherry Orchard* she designed – are infant-sized and scoured green.

I am here for ten days' rest, and immediately I step into Pamela's house I feel lifted. This must also be because of its location: you go to the end of the garden, open a gate and find yourself on Selsey's shingle beach, Bognor Regis far away to your left, Portsmouth to your right. I walk along the causeway and the sea-side houses, bidding good morning to the dog walkers and watching the local frogmen (and one or two frogwomen) pile into a boat to go underwater diving. I come to the bench on the seafront where in 1930 Eric Coates composed the evergreen signature tune for *Desert Island Discs*. Selsey isn't a desert island, just a little town ten minutes' drive from Chichester; but it feels like a haven.

Coates wrote music I grew up with as a war baby: *In Town Tonight*, BBC radio's Saturday night talk show, was heralded by his *In Knightsbridge* and an announcer's voice proclaiming 'We stop the mighty roar of London's traffic to bring you…' Coates also composed the martial music for *The Dam Busters*, my favourite stiff-upper lip tale of World War Two, with plucky and modest Barnes Wallis test-flying his dam-busting bombs by bouncing them along Lake Windermere. I don't know who wrote the signature tune of *Dick Barton – Special Agent*, the BBC's first radio serial, but Dick and his sidekicks Jock and Snowy tied me to the radio week after week, until *The Goons* (music by Ray Ellington), a more grown-up and lunatic programme, ousted it in my affections. Such programmes, and their incidental music, were the soundtrack of my youth. We were the post-war BBC radio generation. And Selsey is suffused with the innocence of that period and that medium.

An Italian friend told Pamela that everyone has a second chance at life, after their first dosage of successes, setbacks and knocks, and that they could only blame themselves if they didn't take the chance. 'Coming here to Selsey was my second chance,' says Pamela. 'I changed from being a victim to being a victor.' The wary patient that I am feels like saying, come on, Pamela, it's a bit too soon to be talking about victory; but she's so radiant and inventive with her new start, I say nothing.

She's built a studio at the end of the garden, where she does the real work of designing plays – plays which, increasingly, she directs as well. There's a model on the worktop for her next piece, *The Marriage*, a Gogol story turned into an opera by Martinů, and which she's transposed to the world of Russian émigrés in 1950s New York. Looking at small-scale models, with their miniature furniture and tiny doll-people always gives me sense of omnipotence, and I feel it again with Pamela's model, an *hommage* to the world of her grandparents. Costume portraits of the principal characters hang from a wire on pegs – indeed the house is pegged throughout, with letters and food-bags and paper decorations hanging from peg teeth, swaying in the air.

During my days in Pamela's diminutive palace-by-the-sea, I realise she and I have trodden similar footsteps through our lives. Born in the same year, 1939, into families with immigrant grand-parents who brought *shtetl* habits and Yiddish to England, Pamela followed me a year later to Planchon's theatre in France, staying even longer, learning even more.

She's very considerate about my need to take things slowly and steadily, asking me if I can handle going to see a play at Chichester Theatre, making sure I take naps when needed and don't over-exert myself. Like me, she has well of energy into which she dips deep. Like me, she is becoming less impulsive about drawing on her energy. Like me, she has a strong entrepreneurial side, and has become a *macher* (a producer and animator, an instigator) as well as a maker. By now, wary of my jack-of-all-trades tendencies, I tell her the story of Tony Harrison – who, when I was commissioned to write Peter Brook's biography, advised me to cut down on my flurry of other activities. 'When the phone rings, and there's an offer to produce another event or write an introduction, just say, "Sorry, that would be one thing too many."'

I tried to make this my mantra; I'm still trying, and sometimes it works. But there's always another side to me that kicks against the constraints of one life in one body and gets up before dawn to write or plan another escapade.

Pamela and I pass in review the many friends we have in common after a career in – and in my case, in and around – the theatre, praising this one's strengths, laughing at that one's shortcomings, indulging in the pleasure of reminiscence and gossip. She keeps coming back to her sense of starting out life as the product of a pocket of Jewish émigré subculture in Newcastle, a Candide in the world of English-ness, wide-eyed at its nuances, its understated rules. This too is familiar to me.

Pamela has just come back from a scenography festival in Prague and before that teaching and directing in Pittsburgh and before that, Venezuela. And now we sit in Selsey, an outpost of English gentility, its silver-haired couples tending the gardens of their retirement homes, many built on a framework of disused railway carriages.

Pamela's arrival here, with her radical and practical interior design – everything within easy hand's reach – and her theatre-maker's know-how, must have been a shock to some of the more staid retirees. But she's now a loved figure, with her red hair and red-and-green-hung house. John, one of the local fisherman, drops in to ask whether any of her 'arty friends' are coming down. 'Yes,' says Pamela. 'Then they'll enjoy this,' says John, and slaps down a sea bass.

Thursday, July 26, 2007

I return to London for the day for a meeting at the hospital to decide whether to go ahead with chemotherapy next week.

The waiting-room at the Rosenheim wing of University College Hospital is crowded with worried people. At the reception desk, the appointments-maker, a stage-door keeper checking people in to their date with fate, admits that he's exhausted, although he only got back from holidays two weeks ago.

I look round the room. Curious phenomenon: there are several couples, but it's hard to tell which one has the illness; both of them look drained.

A man with dark skin, a shock of silver hair and clothes which hang loose on him, enters, sees Jane, and is shocked to find her in an oncology waiting room. He's a former professor at the Institute of Education, another friend and comrade of Jane's past. She says, 'I knocked around with him for a week or two,' and I wonder how close they were. He's relieved when she tells him I'm the one with cancer, not her; she's shocked to see him in such a cavernous condition. He's had cancer of the bowel like me, and a stretch of his colon removed; but unlike me – or unlike me so far, anyway – a secondary cancer was found, in his liver, and he underwent a seven-hour operation.

Of course you expect to run into fellow sufferers in a waiting-room like this, with its squalling little girl and harassed mother and its wife reading out loud to her husband the pamphlet of advice to patients.

I meet my oncologist. The result – he says, opening the sealed envelope – is...inconclusive. Until I have had a further test to determine the extent of damage to my heart, there's no decision. Is this a reprieve? Or a wrist-slap from the gods that govern medicine for daring to imagine I would be able to see ahead? These sudden changes wipe me out.

Rationally, I'd told myself, there could be no expectations that my meeting with Dr Bridgewater would be conclusive, although I'd inured myself to taking chemotherapy for the next six months. But when he announces in a business-like way that the cardiologists want me to take this further test (squirting thallium, a dye, into my heart), all I can do is look at Jane and mutter, 'Well, that makes sense.'

Sense it may make in practical terms; but emotionally, I'm on the rollercoaster again, up and down and tipped into the sea and buffeted by the waves like a cork. Psyched-up for something new, and deposited instead in the waiting-room. It's infuriating, and my fury drains my energy.

I get back to Selsey, to Pamela's house of beauty, and sit still, feeling I've had, in Pamela's mother's words, 'all the stuffing knocked out of me'.

What I haven't been prepared for is the number of e-mailing friends who turn out to have had cancer, or whose wives or partners are undergoing chemo- or radiotherapy now. It feels like stumbling into a forest of cancer-coincidences. Is there a tsunami of cancer out there, a rising flood of cases as relentless as flood waters drowning towns along the Severn, the Avon and the Thames in England this summer?

Has the incidence of cancer risen sharply or am I just running into a web of coincidences? Are the developed countries more prone to it than the developing countries? On the Cancer Research UK website, I find that 'each year 10.9 million people worldwide are diagnosed with cancer; because of the size of its population most of these people (45 per cent) are in Asia'.

The UK, France and Italy each have similar rates of cancer: around a quarter of a million cases each year. Germany has 50 per cent more. The developed world has 46 per cent of world cancer; 'the developing world', 54 per cent.

I note also that:

> the incidence of breast cancer in Japan is much lower than in the USA or the UK. But the incidence of breast cancer in Japanese women living in the USA is the same as for the general population of American women. To doctors, this implies that the causes of breast cancer are probably more closely related to way of life and the environment than to our genetic make up.

'Way of life' means diet and exercise, 'the environment' pollution and pesticides in our food. Issues of age, class, poverty and wealth affect the figures. Are American rates lower because more Americans can afford to join a gym or a health club? Is the steady rise in the figures due to our greater longevity, to 'catching it sooner', a phrase that always implies to me that cancer is a hare, racing ahead of a pack of medical hounds on the dog-track of life?

I am part of a grid – or rather a series of (sometimes contradictory) grids of analysis and interpretation. But they don't play to my feelings of destabilisation, irritation, aggravation and the temptation to give way to passive resignation. To fight these '-ations', I write. Writing is my rage-conduit, my lifeline.

Jane arrives for my final weekend at Selsey. Pamela takes us on a tour of Selsey's caravan park, the biggest trailer-home site I've ever seen, an Orwellian mega-village of identical parked caravans in regulation pastel colours, serviced with security sentinels, far from downtown Selsey but equipped with a leisure centre, a funfair, a school, a mall. Identical avenues of nothingness except for parked cars and shoppers returning to their satellite-saucers and window-boxes. It's like an updated Butlins, frozen in time, totalitarianism lite.

At the sea's edge, an ecological misfortune is taking place: people who bought caravans there so they could skip easily into the sea are now hemmed in with high walls to keep the water out, because the coast is steadily eroding. They look out, not onto waves, but hills of grit.

Wednesday, August 15, 2007

Despite my uncertainties about my medical future, I've not had a bad summer. I'm in good spirits, physically I'm active. Friends who meet me are surprised that I can walk, go to plays and exhibitions and don't look like someone who's been cowering in bed; 'I had not thought death had undone so many.' I would like, however, to be out of this medical limbo, and finally to know whether it's safe for me to go ahead with chemotherapy, or whether its knock-on effect on my heart would be dangerous.

Yesterday I went to University College Hospital and was treated to a 'Thallium scan' of my heart. Thallium, I discover from the invaluable Wikipedia, is 'a very soft and malleable metal and can be cut with a knife. When it is first exposed to air, thallium has a metallic lustre but quickly tarnishes with a bluish-gray tinge that resembles lead.' It has been used for rat poison.

In the scan, a radioisotope is injected, to track blood flow to the heart muscle and the regularity of its movement. It causes the body to emit gamma-rays, which a scanner can detect. Mothers who've had the scan are reassured that the radioactivity it emits is very weak; they will not irradiate their children. I did not glow in the dark.

The scan was administered by a doctor from Sarajevo. He told me he and his family escaped on the last Jewish convoy of trucks and buses out of the city, thanks to his friendship with the head of Sarajevo's Jewish community. What a crossroads this hospital is.

Friday, August 17, 2007

Another appointment with Dr Bridgewater to discuss the results of the scan and the next steps in my treatment. Knowing that he will be dapper, I put on a lightweight suit. He appears in an elegant, loosely-cut, sky-blue shirt.

The upshot of the meeting is that the risk of having chemotherapy on top of my heart condition, and thus causing some kind of heart failure, and the risk of not having it and thus removing a defence against recurring cancer, are more or less equal. So the ball is back in my court. Neither oncologist or cardiologist (whom I am seeing soon) will advise me. I have to choose myself. I know I'm repeating myself, but: if no chemotherapy, a risk of a returning cancer, which would either be treatable with further surgery or radiotherapy, or be (and I quote Bridgewater) 'incurable'. If chemotherapy, a risk of a stroke or heart attack.

I am left with two facts. On the one hand, the fact that I am having a good summer, and feel fine in most respects, not to mention productive as a writer, getting up hours before dawn to add to this text. And my lymph nodes are clear. Both of these factors would point to not doing chemotherapy. Neither of them guarantees that there won't be some malign manoeuvre of my heart or the cancer cells.

So I'm left with a Russian roulette choice, and with nothing but chance and hunch to rely on.

Friends and family are inevitably drawn to give advice: seek a second opinion, go for the chemotherapy, talk to this expert or that specialist. I find myself saying, 'Look, I have every confidence in my consultants, and they know the history and totality of my condition better than any newcomer. Other advice may have been successful with other people, but this is *my* cancer, as personal as my signature.' This will be frustrating for those who think they must *do something*, but in truth the best they can do is be good friends and spend time with me. And the best I can do is to stay calm, not think I'm on some countdown to disaster and try to cram as much as possible into what may be a brief amount of life remaining.

I recall the words of the American poet C K Williams, in his *Of Childhood and the Dark – Danger*:

> Be cautious of your body, which isn't you,
> though neither are you its precise other;
> you're what it feels, and the knowing
> what's felt, yet no longer quite either.
> Your life is first of all what may be lost,
> its ultimate end not to end.

Sunday, August 19, 2007

Yesterday, a rainy Sunday, I spent the day with Monica Vitti. Following Antonioni's death this month, Martin Scorsese wrote a rhapsodic memory piece about seeing *L'Avventura* for the first time, in 1961. He talks about:

> the camera and the way it moved. You never knew where it was going to go, or who or what it was going to follow. In the same way the attentions of the characters drifted: toward the light, the heat, the sense of place, and then toward each other.

I found a DVD of the film, and watched it in spurts through the day. Although I interrupted my viewing of the film, it cast such a spell that it kept calling me back, back to those impassive widescreen black-and-white images, empty islands of towering rock, spume and silence, corridors as long as loss. The film took over my day in a long lingering embrace.

And once more I was transported by Monica Vitti, transported back through time to 1960, when I saw it in a French cinema, in that *annus mirabilis* for the cinema – Buñuel, Godard, Bergman, Rosi, Resnais, changing forever how I looked at moving pictures on a screen. But it was Monica who lifted and touched me, awoke my tenderness and my desire. Her mane of hair; I can imagine it golden, despite the black-and-white image. Her aquiline nose and delicate mouth. Her face so like a Greek actor's mask, a statue of pain. The way Antonioni shot her from behind, and then asked her to spin round in surprise or hurt. The screen like an empty stage, a timelessness into which Monica moved, or from which she departed, leaving a void. When I first saw the film, I wanted to save Monica, to make her happy. I was twenty-one, and romantic, self-exiled from England and unhappily in love, like one of Antonioni's characters striving to know themselves through love-making, shutting their eyes and over-mastered by desire.

I don't want to drool out loud about Monica and me, the perfection of her bare shoulders, her modesty and insecurity, her occasional, touching awkwardness, her – nobility. Suffice it to say that, with Antonioni's elliptical sobriety making me feel calmer and quieter, I was intimate, all through this wet London Sunday, with Monica Vitti. She gave me back the taste of who I was four decades ago.

Heard people on the World Service in the small hours, talking about climate change. They spoke of 'rending the fabric of the universe', which made me think about the fabric of my heart. We don't know the damage we have done to the layers of the atmosphere, nor what worse catastrophe awaits. We can see its signs, but we can't measure how far the damage has gone. So with my heart. I want to see the pictures from the scan of the damage to its muscles, I want the cardiologist to give me her assessment of the heart's future, and how an attack might be staved off. I'm trying to bring the appointment forward, I need to know soon.

I have also been revisiting a favourite film by another great filmmaker who died this month: Ingmar Bergman's *Persona*. It still works the same inexplicable alchemy. As Liv Ullman and Bibi Andersson fight for the upper hand, converge and cross-fade, the physical world is de-materialised, and the screen becomes a stage in which dream and reality melt, like Dalí's droopy watch, softening the contours of our mental categories. On the internet, a Romanian Bergman fan writes that *Persona* is an act of confrontation between Ingmar Bergman and God: the shadow of divine presence, he says, is the Liv Ulmann smile.

Friends e-mail responses to my latest health bulletin, and of course cannot forbear from giving me advice about chemotherapy or no chemotherapy.

'The most alarming thing I've read is your statement about the possibility of "brief life remaining". I've never even heard you suggest that before so I have to assume you are feeling a hopelessness.'

'I'd try a good anti cancer diet instead of chemotherapy.'

'There's a select group of people Death seems to find it extraordinarily difficult to get his grappling hooks into – David Sylvester was one, Harold Pinter is clearly another, and you're an obvious member.'

'At the end of each missive from Perplexed of Crouch End there is a sign. You are probably unaware that it exists since you are unlikely to be a recipient of your own e-mails. Unless, like the fraudster I cross-examined yesterday, you have a variety of e-mail addresses and you send messages to yourself. Anyway, the sign appears after your address. It reads: "No virus found in this outgoing message." Strangely comforting.'

'Why do you mention a "choice"? It seems obvious to me that no one in their right mind (unless they are suicidal – which is not a contradiction in terms) would choose to go for the chemo. There is one certainty: your heart is weak; there is only conjecture as far as your other condition.

'You make me weep. I have no advice – as it seems others have – other than to trust your gut feeling. A combination of that, your intelligence and your good spirits will surely pull you through. Anyway, what would I do if you weren't there? I can't imagine the world without you so you have to hang around.'

Of my friends' messages, this was the one that hit me hardest. It's time to drop the mask of anonymity and talk about the man who sent it: Arnold Wesker, my friend since I was a student, a soulmate, a mirror, a companion, competitor, confidant, someone with whom I argue, someone I forgive, someone who makes me sad, as the prospect of my death makes him weep, it seems.

I also find it hard to imagine life without him. When we first met, at a production I did of *Chicken Soup with Barley* for the Oxford University Labour Club in 1960, he was a leading Royal Court Theatre playwright with *The Wesker Trilogy* and I was an undergraduate stirred by Raymond Williams, Stuart Hall and the New Left. He was cock of the walk in his profession, and I was a student actor and an intellectual, aspiring to get into theatre. From my uncomfortable vantage-point of Oxford's Englishness, it was cheering to see East End Jewish stories and dilemmas on the stage of a theatre in Sloane Square. The realism of these plays' East End Jewish milieu, their immigrant pungency of speech, offhand humour, idealism, sense of struggle, lyrical structure and infectious family closeness, touched more than Jewish audiences. Our reality could have the realism of their reality. Our lives could become the material of theatre.

It was a time when we marched and sang and re-examined every assumption we had encountered, when we welcomed in what we had excluded. The discordant elements of life seemed to be fusing. Tomorrows were singing. His plays caught this hallowing movement of our youth. I was moved by their utopian lyricism; only later did I realise he had an equal awareness of defeat, failure and bitterness.

Then there was the food. He and Dusty were gifted cooks – they'd met in a hotel kitchen – and immensely hospitable. Dinner-parties at his house were frequent, festive, familial and cosmopolitan. I spent Easters with him in Wales, with my girlfriend – we flirted competitively – and later, my first wife. He was like a brother to me; I admired his playwriting, he admired my wide reading.

When he launched Centre 42, his people's arts festivals to bring art and artists closer to working people, I joined his redemptive crusade as a roadie, a poster-sticker and a poetry-reader. The play in each week's festival was Bernard Kops' comedy about a con man, a kind of Jewish Tartuffe; though it spoke of what was to most of its audience an alien culture, it got laughs in Nottingham, Leicester, Wellingborough...

In the middle of Arnold's life, as he seemed to have used up the directly autobiographical source of his plays, his reputation waned, and he suffered several setbacks. His production of his play *The Friends* at the Roundhouse (which he was also seeking to establish as a trades-union-backed centre for people's art) was damaged by a bruising encounter with an actor who sadistically disrupted rehearsals, questioning every note Arnold gave him, nagging and niggling his every remark, on stage and off. It was probably a generous mistake to invite the cast to rehearse in his house in Wales, but he was moved to do so by a messianic desire to fuse art and life, to bring together rehearsal and meals, to make a temporary kibbutz in the Black Mountains. The play was widely dismissed. Critics who, unlike Arnold, had gone to university, called it naïve – an adjective which stuck, as Arnold was cast as a quixotic, misguided idealist.

Arnold seemed to have the capacity to attract hostility. Actors of the Royal Shakespeare Company cast in *The Journalists*, his play set in a newspaper, refused the parts they were offered. The play was a mosaic of tiny scenes and characters, accelerating over a week towards the production of a Sunday newspaper, just as the restaurant kitchen in *The Kitchen*, still his most revived play, accelerated towards the frenzy of dinner time. I thought the actors were as much disappointed by their tiny parts as stirred by a 'people's power' rhetoric that was fashionable in the theatre in the 1970s.

Arnold grew up in a household of East End Jewish Communists who did not practise their Judaism, as I discovered when we tried one year to update the *Seder* service script together and I saw that for all the new 'topical' and 'relevant' inserts, the result lacked the heart – and the infectious folk-tunes – of the original. But, faced with so much hostility, he now began to take on the mantle of the persecuted Jews, and to become fatalistic about anti-Semitism. He rewrote *The Merchant of Venice*, with a more understanding, less villainous, Shylock. 'Jew! Jew! Jew! Jew! I hear the name around and everywhere,' cries his Shylock. 'Your wars go wrong, the Jews must be the cause of it; your economic systems crumble, there the Jew must be; your wives get sick of you – the Jew will be an easy target for your frustration... There's nothing we can do is right.'

He pinned great hopes on the Broadway world premiere of this play, *Shylock,* starring the great American actor Zero Mostel. Mostel died of a heart attack after only one performance on the road. Job could scarcely have had such a succession of bad luck. In Britain, he had the play performed at a regional theatre, but both the National Theatre and the Royal Shakespeare Company turned it down.

When I became head of arts programmes at Channel 4, he needed me to do more for him than I was able to do. For more than a year, I heard nothing from him. I sent postcards and letters; no reply. One Christmas, I ran into him at a party. I'd just come off a plane from New York, and had drunk too much. I blurted out a friend's bewilderment at his silence. He wouldn't explain himself. I insisted he did. He accused me of not doing enough to help his plays get on television. I raised a hand to touch his arm – and found I had left an icing-sugar mark on the sleeve of his black shirt. Two days later he sent me a card, quoting Tynan on *Look Back in Anger*: 'I cannot love anyone who does not love this play.' The truth was, the play in question seemed to me less good than the best of his work. But, foolishly, I did not feel I could be cruel enough to say so. And I also thought there was something histrionic, some playing to the gallery, in quoting Tynan's paean in reference to a minor monologue of his own.

Time passed; after two years we picked up our friendship, as if we needed each other there. Last year he asked me to preface a book of his poems, written across a lifetime. I thought they were painfully honest, but also despairing, mournful for the passing of time and the inroads of age. Through them ran the disappointment of the young man who had once been the apple of his mother's eye. In the lofty style of such prefaces, I called the collection:

> a journey as poignant as a Schubert *Lied*, an extended soliloquy about family, love, ageing, anger, Jewishness… The predominant tone is one of sadness and disenchantment, but never resignation. *All Things Tire of Themselves*, says the poet, but the lifecycle is tirelessly renewed; there is a new child, a change of heart, a fresh season.

When I was writing this, I found a letter he had sent me twenty-five years before, with a poem, 'which I wrote God knows why for God knows whom'.

> I have this fear of ageing maudlin
> Regretting all
> Pleading with my eyes and sighs
> Forgiveness, sympathy
> A worldly understanding
> For the frailty of flesh
> The collapse of passion
> The intellect's senility
> I have this fear.

It conjures up the same picture of a bare ending, as many poems in the book express.

> I fear dismissal from my children
> A wife's weary patience
> The look in friends' eyes
> Remembering, remembering
> The energy, the courage
> The vivid eagerness
> And appetites which were

Once were.

I have this fear.

Reading his poems made me sad for him, a playwright of early success, some of which went to his head, yes, but he sat out the humbling years of refusal that followed, in isolation in a house on a Welsh hillside.

But I couldn't agree with Arnold about Israel, though he had been one of the first to call for a two-state solution. Now, I thought he was, on too little direct experience, back-projecting Holocaust fears to excuse Israel's actions. We clashed about the academic boycott. John Berger had published an article supporting the academic boycott, but carefully arguing that it had to be a matter for each writer or teacher to decide. 'What is important,' he concluded,

> is that we make our chosen protests together, and that we speak out, thus breaking the silence of connivance maintained by those who claim to represent us, and thus ourselves representing, briefly by our common action, the incalculable number of people who have been appalled by recent events but lack the opportunity of making their sense of outrage effective.

When I sent Berger's piece to Arnold, I got an angry response:

> In view of the frightening sight of the Palestinian Hamas Prime Minister ranting before hundreds of thousands like a latter-day Mussolini; and following the declaration last Tuesday from the Iranian President Mahmoud Ahmadinejad to delegates at an international conference questioning the Holocaust that Israel's days were numbered, I think the call for a cultural boycott is ugly, and Berger's argument is spurious and irresponsible.
>
> You know my position. If the Israelis are so terrible then they need the world's cultural genius to illuminate and guide them to the right path. And pragmatically the boycott won't work

because Israel is full enough of its own poets, writers, scientists, and playwrights.

And would you *really* want to sign a boycott that calls upon you not to visit the country?

I am so angry with the way things are going that I want to tell the signatories God damn and blast you all to hell.

How can't you see the dark forces gathering for another Holocaust?

I replied:

If I could think of a better policy to get Israel to stop harassing, uprooting and collectively punishing Palestinians, I'd forget about a boycott. Like you, I think the poet's and playwright's truths may affect a few, but alas a very few, people. And they can be played in Israel to 'unsegregated' audiences – though social and economic disparity excludes most of the 1.2 million Israeli Arabs. So, in true Enlightenment spirit, let plays and films and books circulate. And no, I would not want to accept an embargo on going to Israel – indeed, over the past decade I've been there many more times than you have. And not spent all my time talking to lefties who agree with me.

It's not hard to conjure up the context of this week's horrors, the despicable Teheran conference (with the grotesque anti-Zionist orthodox Jews on the platform with Ahmadinejad spouting his hate-speech). I didn't see the Hamas premier doing what you call his Mussolini act, nor did you, only the TV news report of it, dramatically edited – and isn't Bush just as demagogic, though blessed with TV technology that enables him to act less melodramatically?

The Qassam rockets are a terrible thing for the inhabitants of Sderot, but what one-sided oppression and occupation ultimately triggered them?

Historians like Avi Shlaim show that it was Israel's punitive intransigence that brought Hamas into being. And documentation shows that whenever there was a chance to talk to Palestinians, Israel torpedoed it with targeted assassinations and bombings. I called Avi, as an authoritative historian, to check the facts. The original resolution 181 of 29 November 1947 was indeed rejected by all Arab states. But why, asks Avi, 'should they take back only 55% of their lands?' And he reminds me that on 15 November 1988, the Palestine National Council met in Algeria, accepted by a majority vote Israel's right to exist, and accepted all resolutions relating to the conflict.

I've never believed that an academic or cultural boycott attacks anything but the thinking part of Israel, although my friend Avi Oz, slung out of his post as head of the drama department at Haifa University because one of his students falsely reported him as saying that Israeli soldiers behaved like Nazis, would not necessarily agree.

So if I were to come round to the boycott, it would be a very argumentative kind of support.

Surely you don't want the Israeli intelligentsia to pull up the drawbridge and shout 'ourselves alone'. That may be a besieged Israeli reflex, but to a Diaspora Jew, it seems deeply un-Jewish and isolated.

I don't like reducing our friendship to this cut and thrust. Arnold has been like a brother to me. And writing about him feels a bit like writing an obituary on an unfinished life.

Writing this, I realise I am none too sure what being a brother or having a brother means. It's taken me the best part of a lifetime to see my real brother Lionel for what he is, to recognise among much else that for years he's felt that I never had time for him, while I was always wary about his fits of temper and aggression. It's part of my blur of feelings about family matters, and my alienation from all things familial, to the point that I'm still not sure of the difference between a cousin and a nephew, and never really allowed myself to want children because I couldn't see how they would escape from the blood-thick wrestling of a fractured family.

I can't disentangle my immediate family from my extended family of all Jews. Six years ago, in 2000, when the Second Intifada started, I wrote a kind of open letter to my brother. Playing to the gallery a bit myself, but it's not completely a performance.

A Letter to My Brother on the Eve of Yom Kippur
October 13 2000

When our father was alive, Yom Kippur was for us both the Jewish holiday that on all accounts we had to keep. For me, going to *shul* with Dad on Yom Kippur eventually became more about piety to him than belonging to the congregation. But the emotion and the tunes bit deep, as the clock ticked to the close of the Day of Atonement, and our twilight time for acknowledging misdeeds and qualifying for God's forgiveness ran out.

Today, there's no space for atonement or beseeching. Israel's deeds have been done, with Diaspora Jewry's support, and the crows are coming home to roost like vultures. I hear myself saying to you, 'I can't come to *shul* tomorrow; I don't want to sit with Jews wringing their hands about poor threatened Israel. The only Jews I want to sit with are those who are wringing their minds about how we, how Jews, got like this, got themselves into this stupid, maybe understandable but in the end unforgivable corner.'

David Ben Gurion – who was not blameless, he conceded too much political power to the religious, but then who is blameless in this thing? – Ben Gurion is famously credited with saying in the aftermath of the Six Day War, 'We've won it, now let's give it all back.' That, as my father and his father might have said, was a Jewish *kop* at work. Yes, yes, that's a supremacist remark, claiming that Jewish brains are better than non-Jewish ones. But it's maybe understandable, after generations of being persecuted: you couldn't afford not to be clever in case the Cossacks got you, the Tsarist army conscripted you, the Gestapo or the SS rounded you up. You also needed luck to survive. Howsoever, what Israel has been doing since 1967 lacks some elementary qualities of a Jewish *kop*.

But it also lacks the quality of justice. Isaiah and the Old Testament prophets gave fundamental formulations of righteousness and justice to the Jews and to the world. For the past three decades, a bit more when the right is in power, a bit less when the left has the reins, the Israeli state has replaced them with the practices of an occupying force. As I've been running around this week, goaded by the news bulletins, trying to find a *minyan* of *lamed-vavniks,* about the only statement I could think of us making was, 'Fellow Jews, brothers and sisters, remember Isaiah.' Not much to set against tear gas and tanks and helicopters.

I scour the newspapers for more than reporting, and find David Grossman a distinctive though not exactly heartening Israeli voice. 'Israel may well reach a peace agreement with the Palestinian Authority,' says Grossman. 'But then a much deeper and more threatening confrontation will begin between the Jews and their Arab fellow citizens. Israel has only one way to prevent the bloodshed that such a process would unleash. It must immediately rectify the status of its Arab minority.'

Rectifying the status of (Israel's) 'Arab minority' seems for the time being unthinkable now that thirteen Israeli-Arabs and one Palestinian have been shot within Israel by riot police.

Think about Grossman's phrase 'Arab fellow citizens'. Imagine the almost unimaginable. Imagine that there were no such thing as an Israeli state or a Palestinian state, but a multi-ethnic, secular state of Semites, Jews and Arabs. Each group would have equal democratic and social rights, they would be fellow citizens. Eventually they might become brothers, as you are my brother.

That's it. It's as almost impossible as that. It would mean keeping the religious in their place, ending the idolatrous sanctification of territory just because it is named in the Bible, rethinking 'identity' instead of succumbing to it as fate. It would mean, on 'our side', shaming the dream merchants in Brooklyn and Florida who finance settlements on Arab land into finding better ways of being Jewish than at the expense of other Semites. It would mean Palestinians becoming less apocalyptic and more pragmatic – though the onus lies on our side to act first since we have such a massive superiority of force. It could mean something like a family quarrel about recognising and accepting relatives with whom we have fallen out.

That would be a family worth belonging to. But as it is, brother, and I don't know how you feel on this eve of Yom Kippur, I feel a great distance between me and my Jewish family, the immediate one and the extended one. I will fast tomorrow, as an act of piety to our father and mother. But it's hard to feel fraternity for an Israel which, in the words of Sartre, 'has given up history for the sake of geography'.

But then our uncles would have asked, 'Is Sartre good for the Jews?' The very question takes me back to the Jewishness of our childhood, when it all seemed simple, when you were either for or against the Jews, when we used to laugh at the *Jewish Chronicle* reviewing films and noting that the wardrobe assistant or hairdresser or gaffer was Jewish. Well, that age of Jewish innocence is past.

At nightfall on Yom Kippur 2000, I went to my brother's house to break the fast. My mother opened the door. 'Very disturbing, your letter,' she said. I didn't push it to ask what was disturbing, me or what I described. Soon they arrived: my brother, his Israeli wife, their daughter and her fiancé, their two sons.

After the honeycake and herrings and tea and the fried fish ('I cooked twenty-five pieces,' said my mum, it being a matter of pride and continuity to do so, even at eighty-two), we started shouting about my open letter. It was a pitched battle, loud and interrupted, tortuous and table-thumping, punctuated with the wail, 'Let-me-finish!'

Among the things I heard in my brother's house:

'I agree with what you say, but you come out as anti-Israeli. Some things should be kept in the family.'

'We make all the concessions. They give nothing.'

'They want to drive us all into the sea.'

'After the Holocaust, of course Jews are extra conscious of security.'

'The West Bank Arabs aren't like us; you can't do business with them.'

'You can't trust them. If there's no trust, the only solution is a military one.'

At times, it felt as if people round the table were not speaking but being spoken by knee-jerk sentences, formulaic mottoes. History hardly entered the debate; there was a rush to talk 'realism', legalities and the practicalities of security, on which people suddenly became armchair experts.

My brother, who accepts with pain that there has been injustice and racism in Israel (and he should know – his Yemenite in-laws have suffered their share of prejudice), thought proportional representation was to blame, because it always leads to a coalition in which the religious hold the balance.

'But it's not just mechanics, brother,' I say, 'there's a question of moral will. We have their land, and there's no right of return or recompense. All the new Israeli historians agree: we basically drove them out of their homes in 1948. Of course, the Holocaust forced the issue, but it's still a conflict of two rights, not just poor little Israel against hostile Arab masses.'

August 2007

We go to the Arcola Theatre, to see the last night of Adrian Mitchell's version of Calderón's *The Great Theatre of the World*.

I've known Adrian, poet, playwright and performer, since the Sixties. He set new destinations for me. He has a hotline to childhood; he taps my buried child. He makes word cartoons, makes me laugh and snap my fingers and stomp to his syncopation, then he goes quiet and makes me feel pain, his and the planet's. He comes on like Lennie Bruce and Little Richard. He appears on stage in blue corduroy, with a pair of sky-blue suede shoes.

We used to puff our way up the hill on Hampstead Heath where the kite fliers launch their sails of colour. In our forties, we ran every morning to drive the blues away. 'Time to climb the Acne of Pain.' Now every day he walks the Heath with his lolloping dog Daisy, 'The Dog of Peace'. He says, 'We go there every day, Daisy and me, and pretend we're in the country – we're easily fooled. It's never boring, it changes every day. I'd die for the Heath. I wouldn't kill for it, though.'

To Whom It May Concern, a riveting poem against bombs and cenotaphs and the Vietnam War, with which he stirred a capacity audience in Mike Horovitz's pioneering Poetry Olympics at the Albert Hall in 1965, has lasted through the too many wars since: a durable counting-rhyme to a rhythm and blues beat.

He knows how to write plays for children, which means he can write plays for anyone. He's made plays about Bix Beiderbecke and Hoagy Carmichael, Mark Twain and Jemima Puddleduck. This summer in a field in Kent bigger than two football pitches, Jane and I promenade-watched *The Fear Brigade*, his most ambitious play, performed for and by kids. It was commissioned by the Woodcraft Folk for their Global Peace Camp. Adrian continually breaks out of the cultural compound.

He mines the seam opened by William Blake. His Blake play *Tyger*, about an honest artist trying to survive in a corrupt society, with Adrian's songs and Blake's lyrics set by Mike Westbrook, cracked open the container of Olivier's National Theatre. Quality is not enough; this poet/playwright shows you need fire and subversion; Lorca's *duende*, which 'burns the blood like powdered glass, exhausts, rejects all the sweet geometry we understand, shatters styles.'

For the Arcola Theatre, Adrian has taken Calderón's religious play written for the Spanish Court in an age of faith and made it into a parable of his own faith in humanity and life. Bill Gaskill directs it in the Arcola's sparse space, a former Hackney tailoring sweat-shop, with the afterlife of hard, bent-back labour in its walls. A young cast scamper on, wearing skull-masks and leotards painted with skeletons, like the death-dancers I saw in San Juan Bautista, California twenty years back, celebrating *Dia De Los Muertos*, the Day of the Dead.

In the Gaskill/Mitchell version, Calderón's Catholic-tinged piece harks back to its Aztec origins, in which death is not a negation of life. In San Juan Bautista, skulls made of sugar were heaped on the graves of the dead, and eaten by their surviving relatives. A rough street band got us shuffling round the town in the hot sun, tequila was consumed in generous qualities, and a cabaret of misfortune, *El Fin Del Mundo* was performed in a big barn. At the Arcola, there's the same defiantly joyful spirit. Rewards and punishments are handed out by the great Director In The Sky to the Beggar, the King, the Rich Man and the Peasant. The joker in the pack – or rather, its tragedy – is the corpse of a stillborn baby who never even made it to this world. For Adrian, this baby is 'the rock in the play. How could God let this happen?'

Adrian's text is full of images of the plenitude and brevity of the world.

> My darling planet, my darkling planet,
> You steal your light and heat from my heavens.
> Your millions on millions of beautiful flowers
> Reflect my millions of stars,
> But their glowing, petalled galaxies
> Are rooted in earth, and drink from the earth
> And return to the earth when they fade into death.

I feel closer to his images of death than I would have done before this brush with last things in my own life.

> This is the cradle, shaped to receive.
> This is the grave by which you leave.

I've found a literary companion, Samir el Youssef. We meet several times a week in the Spiazza Italian Food Hall, which has lit up Crouch End's town hall square. I met him a couple of years ago at a launch for *Gaza Blues*, a book of short stories by an Israeli writer Etgar Keret and a novella by Samir, who is a Palestinian living down the road in a street I used to inhabit. Among shelves of seductively packaged Italian products, we engage in writers' café talk. I'd liked the cool irony of his fiction and enjoy talking to him. We usually start with writing. How's it going? How far have you got? He encourages me to take risks in my writing. 'Don't be too English, Michael. Your ancestors came from the Mediterranean. Go for broke.'

Samir was born 43 years ago in Rashidia refugee camp in Southern Lebanon and has been living in London for seventeen years. He's robustly built, with a shock of curly hair and bright black eyes. He likes doing imitations of upper-class English speak: 'old chap', 'old fruit'. He has a big laugh.

He managed to get out of the camp and go to 'what they call a university' in Sidon. But the Lebanese civil war made life dangerous for Palestinians. 'How can a country which can't be hospitable to its own people be hospitable to Palestinians?' he asks me. He left the country and went to Cyprus, and from there to London, where he studied philosophy at Birkbeck College. He made a living as a journalist for the Arabic press, and started writing fiction and essays. Now he writes in English, a writer transplanted like Joseph Conrad – only weighted with the Israel/Palestine conflict, on which everyone he meets in London has an opinion. He's scathing about well-meaning but under-informed English liberals, but equally hard on Utopian Palestinian exiles dreaming of return. His novel *The Illusion of Return* and his stories are populated by Palestinians weaving theories of political redemption in smoky West London cafés. Conversations which might have taken place among Russian exiles in Zurich before the Revolution, or German refugees in Swiss Cottage in the 1930s.

Samir has a wife in Sidon. They see each other periodically, there or here, at present for little more than two months a year. I discover we share the same birthday, so we arrange a joint celebration, at a little Greek restaurant. There are ten of us, his friends and mine. Later he tells me how unsociable he is: this was the largest number of people he's met at one time. He doesn't like parties full of strangers; I've seen him getting aggressive and argumentative on such occasions. Mostly he spends his days writing, in a room he rents from an old woman he cares for. Evenings, he reads determinedly – classic novels and recently Shakespeare, whom he reads cover to cover in little editions with no footnotes on the pages to spoil the text. I keep trying to get him to come out and see Shakespeare in performance, but theatre-going seems too much of a social event. Literature is his homeland.

I've gradually realised that Samir is, profoundly and philosophically, the most exiled person I know. In *The Illusion of Return* I find out why. The narrator meets another exile friend, Ali, passing through London on his way back to Lebanon. Ali talks about Bruno, an old Jew he has met who believes that returning to one's place of birth, nostalgia for roots, homecoming, is meaningless.

> 'He was not sure it was right for Jews to go to Palestine!'
> 'Didn't he believe in his right of return to the promised land?' I asked seriously, and I was surprised that I asked the question in such a manner. I had meant it to be sarcastic, but it came out as a serious question.
> 'What? Poor Bruno,' Ali exclaimed, 'he didn't believe in the right to return anywhere.'
> 'Bruno didn't think that it was possible for people to return,' Ali explained. 'He believed that people only moved on; even when they went back to the place of their birth and early life they were only moving on.'

It's a pitilessly clear-eyed position, and one that Samir, for all his high spirits, espouses. His exilic outlook makes my own alienation look small. But he's in his first-generation diaspora (the second, if you count his parents' 1948 expulsion from Israel as the first); I'm a third-generation, displaced Russian/Polish Jew. We have shared undertones and a fate in common as we talk among the Illy coffee and *amaretti* at Spiazza.

Saturday, August 25, 2007

Twelfth Night at Chichester.

Michael Feast hits the Chichester stage like an uncaged bird. His Feste cracks the play open; he brings into its rueful comedy of love misplaced and twins mistaken not only wit, speed and virtuosity, but a mental agility, a rage and a madness that make the principal characters' delusions look small. More than any Feste I've seen, Feast, all quicksilver questioning and cleansing scorn, turns the world of sense and decorum upside down. 'Nothing that is so, is so.'

Feast is like a sparrow, pecking up cues for wordplay and puns, racing round the stage, shifting pace, tempo and direction, turning on a sixpence, letting loose his skittering mind. He's a world away from the Festes of convention: the poignant Watteau clowns, picturesque Harlequins or, more recently, the Archie Rice-like music-hall hoofers. Feast seizes the anger under the laugh-lines and pay-offs. Delivering Feste's sad songs of youth that will not endure, of death that awaits us all, he becomes a natty and waspish nightclub star, a Las Vegas bill-topper. His Feste is also a linguistic philosopher. 'Words,' he says, 'are very rascals... Words are grown so false I am loath to reason with them.' 'Art thou not the Lady Olivia's fool?' replies Viola. 'No indeed, sir, I am indeed not her fool but her corrupter of words.'

I've known Feast since he arrived at the National Theatre in 1974, playing Ariel and struggling with his inner demons. He's been the Duke in *Measure for Measure*, Mephistopheles in Marlowe's *Faustus* and later Goethe's Faust, Foster in Pinter's *No Man's Land* and Hermes in Tony Harrison's film *Prometheus*, scathing about what humanity has done with the gift of fire.

He's adept at hanging fractionally on line-endings, plucking keywords out of a line for an audience's inspection, accelerating athletically, injecting blocks of silence into the flow of sounds. He brings fastidiousness to Feste's commentary on his own choice of words: 'My lady is within, sir, I will construe to them whence you come. Who you are and what you would are out of my welkin. I might say "element" but the word is overworn.'

His show-biz dance-steps and his polished patter are powered by madness, a laser-beam of lunacy which takes him through the surface of things to their core. Dressed up as the priest Sir Topas to torment the humbled Malvolio in his dark cell, he swaps voices with his 'real' self as Feste – much as Edgar plays with Lear's credulity, switching from 'Poor Tom' to his own voice. You sense the comedian dancing on the precipice of reality and appearance and the acts that mortals adopt.

In the National Film Archive Michael discovered a two-minute clip of his great-grandfather doing his music-hall act. He adds to this discovery the routines of live entertainers and stoic clowns, from his Buster Keaton-like straw boater to his Crazy Gang soft-shoe shuffle and his Danny Kaye impishness – though Danny Kaye was more of a Sweet Fool than Feast's Feste.

Live theatre has been my occupation and my touchstone for forty years. I wrote a book in defence of live theatre in the digital age, *theatre@risk*. Simon Callow reviewed it in *The Guardian*. 'It would not be quite accurate to describe him as central to the theatre,' he wrote;

> He acknowledges as much himself: it has been his profession, he says, but not his vocation. Kustow is by temperament a fan, a passionate, informed, articulate fan; by profession an enabler... who facilitates, encourages and promotes, but ever present is the sense of the nose pressed against the window.

Perhaps people like me who are hopelessly in love with theatre, to such a point that they can't turn it into a career, for whom it's a vocation never to be fully realised, are always going to feel this way.

I marvelled at actors when I was young, wanted to be an actor, but there were obstacles – my stammer, the conviction drummed into me that it wasn't a real job, like being a lawyer, doctor or accountant.

I would have been an actor if I could.

Peter Brook and I were sitting around at the Aldwych Theatre one day, while Peter Hall was rehearsing Gogol's grotesque master-piece *The Government Inspector*. One of its many comic inventions is the eerie pair of near-twins, Bobchinsky and Dobchinsky. Gogol describes them as:

> short little fellows, strikingly like each other. Both have small paunches and talk rapidly, with emphatic gestures of their hands, features and bodies. Dobchinsky is slightly the taller and more subdued in manner. Bobchinsky is freer, easier and livelier. They are both exceedingly inquisitive.'

'You know, Michael,' said Peter, 'you and I could play those parts.'

Friday, August 31, 2007

Yesterday I had the appointment with the cardiologist.

I've been speculating on the phrase 'the horns of a dilemma,' from which I seem to be suspended. It's a no win/no lose situation: do chemotherapy, and I may risk a stroke or heart attack; don't do chemotherapy, and the cancer may have a better chance of recurring. On the internet, I find a site called World Wide Words, written by Michael Quinion, and read that:

> the original *dilemma* in rhetoric was a device by which you presented your opponent with two alternatives; it didn't matter which one he chose to respond to – either way he lost the argument. When you did this to your opponent you were said to present two horns to him, as of a bull, on either of which he might be impaled.

Exactly.

The night before the appointment, I noted that my heart was beating faster than usual, and I felt a kind of dull apprehensiveness. I had planned to spend the evening watching a Bergman film, *Cries and Whispers*, but decided that this was too sombre, and chose instead Woody Allen's *Manhattan* – only to find, of course, that it features an argument about Bergman's movies. Achingly funny as when I first saw it, a combination of freewheeling verbal wit and impassively calm shooting and editing.

I stop the film and call people I'm close to. First Orna, to whom I was married for twenty years.

'Decision time about my cancer treatment is upon me,' I say. 'And I spent this morning at my mother's house with my brother, packing up the last things before the house is sold next week. This day feels like a crossroads in every way.'

Then I call Jane's brother Andy, in Sheffield, then her other brother Tim, in Trieste. One way or another, this is telling me that when the heat is on, it's still family I turn to.

My appointment, at 8.30am, is with Dr McEwan. I had learned that Dr McEwan was a woman, and had figured she'd be like Geraldine McEwan: tall, wide-eyed, bird-like. The cardiologist McEwan turns out to be quick, voluble and less angular than the actress McEwan. I spend an hour with her, which includes a brief tutorial on atrial fibrillation, my condition, an examination from top to toe, and a scrutiny on the computer screen of the results of my heart scan and echo cardiogram. Dr McEwan scrolls through black and white images of my heart, visual slices on different planes, from which I can see a distended left atrium and a calcified aorta. My bowel is a big soft-looking sack, in which faeces are lodged. Valves, arteries and veins tap into the heart. 'The danger,' says Dr McEwan, 'is that with a weakened pumping action, bits of blood will collect in crevices, coagulate and could become a clot.'

I tell her I've realised in the past week that my biggest fear, even more than a return of the cancer, is to have a stroke, and be partially paralysed or lose my speech. She nods, encouragingly; I feel tear-ducts stirring as I say this.

Her final assessment, which she will circulate to my oncologist, my surgeons and my GP, is that my heart is not so damaged that chemotherapy would have a dangerous knock-on effect. She's not advocating a course of action, just telling me the state of play in my chest. So I'm still left hanging from those horns of the dilemma.

She tells me that there is a study of clinical trials in which patients who had elected to have chemotherapy were compared with those who'd declined to have it, and encourages me to call the oncologist and get the statistics.

She has been sufficiently positive about the state of my heart and about the fact that the lymph nodes around the perforated colon showed no signs of infection that I'm beginning to feel I should refuse chemotherapy. If I am closely monitored with blood tests and scans in aftercare, it should be possible to catch any cancer reappearance at an early stage, and then do chemotherapy if necessary – or radiotherapy or surgery again.

I thank her, we shake hands, and I ask her if I can call her Jean. 'I prefer Dr McEwan, and I'll call you Mr Kustow,' she says. 'I tell my students to avoid calling their patients by their first names.' I respect this; it keeps a structure between patient and doctor. Very classical in its formality,

I walk back to the bus through University College and Gordon Square, from where I call Bernard Kops; Jane is unreachable on the train back from the Lakes with the grandchildren. Kops is upbeat, as so often. 'I'm eighty, and I've decided that so much could go wrong that there's no choice but to live fully in the here and now. So I've invented a new philosophy: Now-ism. You're a Now-ist, too, Michael. I spell it N-A-O-I-S-T.'

At home, I call my GP Dr Kaz, to report. When I tell him of my fear of having a stroke, it turns out that his mother had one at the age of forty-nine, and couldn't move or speak. 'But,' he adds, 'taking chemotherapy will hammer those little cancer cells into oblivion.' Yes, I say, but if it's at the price of a stroke... And then I say what I've been feeling for weeks: that deciding to do chemotherapy feels like a macho, assertive response, whereas deciding not to do it feels... wimpish by comparison. It isn't, of course, it's just a choice, but a choice made in a culture where intervention, *doing something rather than doing nothing*, is the sovereign virtue.

I tell Dr Kaz that I'm going to see a dietician who specialises in heart cases, and that I've been keeping at bay all my friends' well-meaning offers of complementary medicine, special diets and supplements. 'Quite right,' he says. 'Even taking vitamins could upset the chemical balance of your existing medications.' So, rebellious in many fields, but conservative in this one, I'm going to decide that I will go for aftercare monitoring instead of chemotherapy. Whatever I may learn from my oncologist about the data of the clinical trials will make no difference. There's a danger anyway of information overload. Enough is enough.

The other thing I do, which is a kind of wager on the future, is to fix on November 18, my birthday, as the deadline by which I have to have completed the next draft of my play. Having such a goal is part of my bid to stay alive, and not to fret needlessly about the fate of my body.

Chapter Six:
ANGER AND HOPE

Monday, September 3, 2007

Jonathan Miller debates atheism with John Gray at the British Library – or rather debates the more aggressive motion 'Science Makes Religion Redundant'. Because of a Tube strike, the start is delayed, and Jane and I sit in the auditorium and watch the audience come in, with their kindly faces, silver hair and uncertain gait (they probably see us in the same way). The reading-rooms where I work are also packed, predominantly with young people. And the high lobby, with its epic R B Kitaj tapestry, *If Not, Not,* is a lively human crossroads. So why is tonight's audience so elderly? What have I got against the middle-aged anyway?

Jonathan, whom I've known on and off, in and out of theatres, tucks his long legs around the chair and gazes out, at once beady and gloomy. John Gray, Professor of European Thought at LSE, looks like an academic out of a David Lodge novel: rimless glasses, tweed jacket and tidy posture compared with Jonathan's sprawl.

Gray has just published *Black Mass – Apocalyptic Religion and the Death of Utopia,* a denunciation of the cruelties practised in the name of religious faith, and of the horrors wrought by secular utopian ideologies. His main thesis is that there is no such thing as secular thought: behind every secular scheme lies a religious pattern. Even the Marxist belief in a redemptive finale to history is Messianic at heart, says Gray.

Jonathan argues in a very different and, it must be said, more entertaining, way. For a start he is more autobiographical. He admits to never having had a religious thought in his life. No intimations of a Mighty Being at an early age; 'There was just a blank where others had belief'. He doesn't like being labelled an atheist, for that would imply a *theos* in which to disbelieve. He says he started out as 'an inarticulate disbeliever', only becoming articulate when he studied medicine and began to think scientifically.

Jonathan attacks the word 'spirituality', comparing it with 'lighter fuel that spills everywhere when the lighter is broken'. He gets a lot of mileage – and laughs – from this analogy, like a comedian using a punchline. His speech is both philosophically knotty – he quotes Thomas Nagel and a Wittgensteinian honesty underpins his sentences – and pure cabaret.

But then Jonathan Miller is an artist as well as a scientist, a performer as well as a thinker. He pauses to consider 'embodiment', a concept which fascinates him, as well it might, given his elongated body – and the stammer which he negotiates by sidestepping into wider vocabularies with words that don't start with dangerous consonants.

A former stammerer myself, I know how aware one becomes of the disparity between the mind and the body, the desire to communicate and the recalcitrance of tongue, palate and lips.

I admire Jonathan as a 'non-Jewish Jew', to use Isaac Deutscher's invaluable phrase. I remember a conversation with Jonathan at Harvard when I was working there in 1981 and invited him to lecture about theatre. Afterwards, we got on to talking about feeling Jewish and yet keeping a distance from tribal allegiances. I asked him what he thought about Jerusalem. Wasn't he touched by its enveloping atmosphere of – I confess I used the word – spirituality? I got a vehement reply. 'I can't stand the place. People rocking backwards and forwards mumbling prayers at the Wailing Wall, slaughtering infidels, beating their heads bloody against the stones.'

Jonathan is the very type of what Stalin called 'the rootless cosmo-politan' – restless, never satisfied, the archetypal insubordinate spirit, never likely to merge into a community or a congregation. His great friend Susan Sontag shared this drive to challenge and contest the certitudes of faith, aesthetics or politics. Neither of them has ever quite lost the need to be recognised as the cleverest in the class. Have I?

Jonathan Miller belongs to that central tradition of the best in Jewish culture – indeed, in world culture – being produced by Bad Boys and Bad Girls, not by unthinking, corporate identity.

In a 1958 lecture, *The Message of the Non-Jewish Jew*, which became the title of the last book he wrote, Isaac Deutscher surveyed the legacy of Spinoza, Heine, Marx, Rosa Luxemburg, Trotsky and Freud.

> Have they anything in common with one another? Have they perhaps impressed mankind's thought so greatly because of their special 'Jewish genius'? I do not believe in the exclusive genius of any race. Yet I think that in some ways they were very Jewish indeed. They were *a priori* exceptional in that as Jews they dwelt on the borderlines of various civilisations, religions and national cultures. They were born and brought up on the borderlines of various epochs. Their minds matured where the most diverse cultural influences crossed and fertilised each other. They lived on the margins or in the nooks and crannies of their respective nations. They were each in society and yet not of it, of it and yet not in it. It was this that enabled them to rise in thought above their societies, above their nations, above their times and generations, and to strike out mentally into wide new horizons and far into the future.

These heroic dissenters form a Jewish Diaspora tradition. I do my best to keep company with them.

Tuesday, September 18, 2007

I thought I'd made my mind up and decided not to go forward with chemotherapy. But this week my mobile rang. It was the Registrar of University College Hospital oncology department. 'We've received a letter from your cardiologist saying that there would be no risk of an effect on the heart and that it's safe to go ahead with chemotherapy, so we've booked you a slot in ten days' time, if you want to take it up.'

The heartbeat quickens. Have I really made the right decision? Am I needlessly laying myself open to the recurrence of the cancer?

'What's the name of the cardiologist who wrote this letter?' I ask.

He mentions the name of a man I've never seen. I was seen by a Scottish woman doctor, the formidable Dr McEwan. I point this out. Is he sure the letter applies to me? Is some other patient awaiting a diagnosis which has been sent to me by mistake?

He retreats apologetically. I ask him to take me through the percentage benefits I would have if I took chemotherapy. It would offer some reassurance. But the figures are confusing, and don't seem to tally with the ones I've already been quoted. I fix to see the oncologist in a few days' time, put down the phone and look round the garden feeling winded.

It's a bright afternoon with blazing sun. We're sitting with Julian and Linda in the garden of the Chelsea Arts Club. Julian has just opened a show of his paintings of Tibetan mountains and Lake District quarries, and we're celebrating in this haunt of steady-drinking bohemians, a last outpost of the Soho of the 'fifties. Though his subjects are mountains and quarries, they're far from being landscape or topographical paintings. Julian has gazed so long and so deeply at rocks and streams that they have become elemental presences in his work, impassive monsters shouldering their way into the frame, threatening to burst out of it. He seems to have captured the forces of geology itself; the surface erupts, cracks like a rock face.

At the private view, I was irritated by the silhouettes of other viewers coming between me and the pictures. They demand uncluttered concentration.

Jane and I walk to the bus back home. I'm seething again. Just when I thought I'd got rid of the need to think about whether to chemo or not to chemo, back it comes again, taking up precious mental space and emotion.

Next day I write to all my consultants.

> On Friday I received a call from the Registrar of the oncology department. He informed me that they had received a letter from the cardiologist, who has said there was now no obstacle from their point of view about proceeding with chemotherapy. Nothing untoward about this – except that the name of the signatory of this letter – Dr Swanton – was not that of the cardiologist I actually saw, Dr McEwan. This mistake creates doubt and uncertainty.
>
> The Registrar then ran through the percentages involved if I took chemotherapy. I summarise, I hope correctly: 'a 15 per cent increase in the chances of cancer not recurring; and an improvement of up to 4 per cent in my chances of living for another five years'.
>
> Meanwhile, who is the mystery consultant who signed the letter and who I have never met?

Thursday, September 20, 2007

When I walk into Dr Bridgewater's office, he has put up on the screen the study comparing cancer patients who have taken chemotherapy with those who haven't. A graph indicates that there's only a five per cent benefit. The risk of getting a stroke because of the chemotherapy is roughly the same. So much I knew already. My cancer has been classified as T4 0/21 Mo, which means it has punctured the wall of my colon, but hasn't spread to other organs. Dr Bridgewater apologises for the mistake about the cardiologist's letter – 'It was PP'd incorrectly' – runs through side-effects (fatigue, dry mouth, diarrhoea, hair-loss). I ask him to give me his opinion of the seriousness of my cancer. 'Not the worst case,' he says, and then asks me what I want to do about chemotherapy.

Now I feel I've got the real data. 'I don't want it,' I say. 'But I do want regular monitoring so any recurrence can be caught early.'

'We'll give you standard surveillance,' he says. For the first time he cracks something resembling a smile. 'I think it's a good decision,' he says, writing a note in my file.

I step out with Jane into the Bloomsbury air. I have a sense of relief and a spring in my step, now that I've been endorsed by the doctor, having fought my way back to the clinical studies, the experimental basis of the statistics with which I've been battered.

Russell Square looks idyllic in the late sun. A man's playing a flute to his girlfriend and to a squirrel, who hops appreciatively. I say goodbye to Jane and sit for an hour outside the café, watching young women trot past and young men chat up young women.

In the evening, I go to *Fragments*, five short Samuel Beckett plays that Peter Brook has mounted in the Young Vic's studio theatre, with Kathryn Hunter, Jos Houben and Marcello Magni, members of Theatre de Complicite who know each other's work inside out. They cut visual and verbal shapes in the empty space, outlines against the cement back wall. An abstract, slowly changing grid of light provides visual punctuation between the pieces; reminds me of the segments in a Rothko painting. *Fragments* is a blackly humorous vaudeville of living, waiting and dying. Sobering, but strangely bracing too.

Brook's programme note mirrors many things I'm feeling, about life, about theatre:

Today, with the passage of time, we see how false were the labels first stuck on Beckett – despairing, negative, pessimistic. Indeed, he peers into the filthy abyss of human existence. His humour saves him and us from falling in, he rejects theories, dogmas, that offer pious consolations, yet his life was a constant, aching search for meaning.

He situates human beings exactly as he knew them in darkness. Constantly they gaze through windows, in themselves, in others, outwards, sometimes upwards, into the vast unknown. He shares their uncertainties, their pain. But when he discovered theatre, it became a possibility to strive for unity, a unity in which image, sound movement, rhythm, breath and silence all come together in a single rightness. This was the merciless demand he made on himself – an unattainable goal that fed his need for perfection. Thus he enters the rare passage that links the ancient Greek theatre through Shakespeare to the present day in an uncompromising celebration of one who looks truth in the face, unknown, terrible, amazing…

Tony Graham calls. When I tell him I'm fasting for Yom Kippur out of 'piety', there's a bit of a silence. 'Do you understand what I mean by piety?' I ask. 'Yes, it's the thing that saints do.'

'But I don't mean that, I mean something between reverence and memory. The loyalty we owe our parents.'

Before I dissolve into misty-eyed, all-forgiving sentiment, I remind myself of the battles I have fought with my parents. The conflict with my father was easy to understand: a full-frontal, head-on collision of wills. With my mother it was much harder, because she was a more elusive presence: an insidious controller. Being or playing being a victim is often the most powerful form of control over others.

She was an expert. With a sigh she could take your *kishkes* out. I use *kishkes,* the Yiddish word for 'guts' or 'intestines', the part of my body where the cancer has been at work, because today is Yom

Kippur, the Jewish Day of Atonement. I don't know whether I have anything to atone for; some remorse perhaps, but no action or refusal to act that replays itself in my mind and makes me squirm. But I'm going to *shul*, to synagogue, with Sandy Lieberson, whose daughter's *batmitzvah* I attended, and whose new-found Jewishness has brought Sandy and his non-Jewish wife Sarah Parkin back 'into the fold', though Sandy never struck me as a sheep who had gone astray.

Anyway I'm going, and around noon I will say a prayer in remembrance of my mother, or simply as a marker to remember that she died a little over a year ago.

September 2007

Channel 4 is marking its twenty-fifth anniversary, with a season of arts programmes at the Barbican Centre. After twenty-five years in which television has been multi-channelised, Murdoch-ised and simply got more strident, the first wave of commissioning editors is asked which Channel 4 arts programmes we consider most 'iconic.' Jan Younghusband, my successor as arts commissioning editor, says there's no comprehensive list of commissioned programmes, so from memory I dredge up a list, an inevitably invidious choice:

Tony Harrison, 'V'   An angry, elegiac film-poem about the desecration of the poet's parents' tomb by hooligans, the miner's strike, the skinhead inside us all, put into images by Richard Eyre. It provoked a tabloid storm because Tony liberally sprinkled four-letter words in the mouth of his skinhead character. CHANNEL SWORE headlined the *Daily Mail*.

Pina Bausch, '1980'   A two-hour dance theatre piece, a surreal succession of scenes and images of love and death, *put out in primetime*. A puzzled viewer rang in to say he didn't understand what was happening but he hadn't been able to drag himself away from it for the past hour.

'A TV Dante' The painter Tom Phillips and the film-maker Peter Greenaway transformed Dante's poem (which Phillips also translated anew) into multi-layered video, combining hand-made graphics and images from heart-scans and newsreels with Sir John Gielgud as Virgil and Bob Peck as Dante.

Peter Hall / Tony Harrison, 'The Oresteia' Aeschylus' trilogy about war, violence and retaliation, directed by Peter Hall and performed by a company in masks, which were often more eloquent than the unmasked faces of television personalities. Three hours of television in alliterative verse.

'The Mahabharata' Peter Brook's re-creation on film of his six-hour stage version of the Indian saga. Apart from its other virtues, it was a pioneer example of 'integrated casting', with a cast of Indian, English, Japanese, Italian and Polish actors.

'About Time' Mike Dibb's six-part documentary essay on the varieties of time, from menopausal time to the chartered time of the stock exchange, by the director who, with John Berger in *Ways of Seeing*, revolutionised the television presentation of art and arguments about.

'Monuments and Maidens' Marina Warner and Gina Newson's exploration of the mythology of femininity, from Joan of Arc to statues of naked women symbolising virtue.

Hermione Lee, 'Book 4' A thoughtful series about books and literature, presented by the biographer of Virginia Woolf, which failed to attract the audience it deserved. Since then, there has been no regular programme on television dedicated solely to books and reading. Maybe radio does it better.

Michael Nyman, 'The Man who Mistook his Wife for a Hat' An original opera based on Oliver Sacks' neurological case study, written and directed by Chris Rawlence, which drew forth some of Nyman's most affecting music.

'Voices' A late-night debate series about art, politics and ideas, chaired first by Al Alvarez and then by Michael Ignatieff, and produced by Udi Eichler. Participants included Susan Sontag, John Rawls, Octávio Paz and George Steiner. With its Persian-carpet-hung walls, it became the egg-heads' favourite television rendezvous. Egg-heads have rights too.

Our successes with such programmes were never huge in ratings terms, but we saw our audience as a mosaic of minorities. Looking at the list, I think how different it was twenty-five years ago. In 1982, starting a new channel from scratch, with the BBC going through a dip in confidence, we had money to spend, yawning slots to fill and a crusading energy. The channel's brief, was to do work of a different kind to the other channels, to represent whole swathes of British life that never got onto the small screen. I was trying to commission, not television about the arts, not art televised, but art television – television inflected by art and artists, programmes as full-hearted, sharp-minded and kitsch-averse as a good poem, painting or performance.

When I joined the channel, I was greeted by my chief executive Jeremy Isaacs with the words, 'Are you sure you're being avant-garde enough, Michael?' Which television supremo would say such a thing today?

In the channel's early years, we regularly included the arts in the 7pm news, not to mock avant-garde pranks but to treat them as part of our reality just as much as politicians or floods. Now they are ghettoised into often marginal arts slots, the same as on every other channel. The channel at its outset ventured into the battleground of ideas and the debate about the place of culture itself, addressing the whole person, not just the arts customers and consumers. What is culture, it asked, in our society and in a globalised world? No sign of that now on today's Channel 4, and not much on any television channel; reflection is left to radio.

The first art television programme to be screened on Channel 4 in 1982 wasn't even listed in the schedules. When we began, there wasn't enough advertising to fill the breaks. The blanks were usually filled by the advertising sales department with trailers or anodyne music and stills.

The poet Christopher Logue and I concocted the idea of 'poetry shorts' – programmes of a minute or less in which Logue, in his corncrake voice, read some of the best poems in the English language while the screen showed the text of the poem, in black and white. The series, which re-invented the song sheet, was called *Edible Gold;* its miniature programmes were slotted unbilled and unannounced into the empty commercial spaces. We didn't want an unctuous or smart-arse continuity announcer setting them up. Unprepared, viewers ran into poems by Blake, Pound or Adrian Mitchell. In a tiny way, we reintroduced surprise into the fabric of television.

Today the 'media landscape' (a phrase much beloved by media pundits, of whom there weren't many in 1982) has changed beyond recognition. Rupert Murdoch's systematic raids on the system, together with the proliferation of channels and 'platforms', have segmented the audience into sports-lovers, news junkies, movie buffs, porn addicts. The public vocation of television to speak to a broad general audience, the Reithian imperative to inform and educate as well as divert and entertain – admirable, for all their earnestness – have been eroded.

Channel 4 has not been immune to the new ethos, succumbing to the worldwide epidemic of reality television with *Big Brother,* which is voyeuristic, pseudo-democratic and cheap to make. Such programmes on all channels have been convicted and fined for defrauding viewers on their phone-ins. The BBC is wriggling on the floor again like a beached whale, with its license fee cut, its overpaid presenters and meddling layers of middle management. So much television has become a parade of clownish eccentrics. Chefs become stars, chat-show hosts literary arbiters. Turn on and you are more than likely to fall on a show in which bossy Sloane Rangers teach bewildered ordinary folk how to make over their house, buy a retirement residence on the Costa Brava or dress properly. Off-screen announcers sport a tabloid chirpiness or regional accents to signify authenticity. What happened to 'public service' television, or more simply to public television? It's getting harder to distinguish the programmes from the commercials. Is television delivering programmes to viewers, or audiences to advertisers? Where is the Hogarth to depict this Bedlam of the media?

The market rules, Murdoch's market, Thatcher's market, the neoliberal marketisation of practically everything. We used to be proud of our 'public sphere'; now it's shrunk to a chain of marketplaces. As the border between private and public has become porous, a shrill individualism has moved in.

I know I get tetchy and preachy about these reversals, but I've been around long enough to see the steady retreat from worthwhile goals.

Tuesday, October 2, 2007

Jane comes down to my study and we watch Renoir's *La Règle du Jeu* on DVD. Such zest, such *élan* in the playing; such fluid shooting and musical editing. What an ensemble of prodigious players: the complaisant husband (Marcel Dalio) and the poacher (Julien Carette) who tries to snaffle the gamekeeper's wife act with their whole bodies. Renoir draws on the culture of Beaumarchais and Feydeau, their light-as-air comedy. The film is a fresco of a depleted class, about to give in to the Nazi occupation, which came a year after the film was made; and of their servants, playing their assigned parts in the game of privilege and class, their self-esteem leased from their masters.

I murmur as the gamekeeper suffers yet another rejection from his flighty wife, a coquettish maidservant. I laugh at the bitter playfulness of Renoir's gay dance of death, its emblematic carnival toys pirouetting as mechanically as the effete count whose playthings they are. And, for all its vigour, it's so understated, so humane.

The film ends. Jane gets up to depart upstairs, where she sleeps, because I wake in the small hours. This illness gets everywhere.

She opens the front door to leave. I stand still, being left.

'Are you okay?' she asks.

'I feel sad,' I say.

There's a silence as our eyes meet.

'It's hard, I know,' she says. And, as if in slow motion, goes.

It began so differently.

Bristol, 1961.

Saturday night, the end of a week-long 'People's Arts Festival'. After folksong in the pubs, paintings in supermarkets, plays in school halls, comes the week's finale – The Big Band Ball. This week it's in the vast hangar of British Aerospace in Filton, Bristol. We've brought our artists and scenery to Wellingborough, Leicester, Nottingham, Hayes; I've been a roadie and a performer, humping lights and loudspeakers, pitching events from soapboxes on street corners, reading Brecht poems in factory canteens. Arnold Wesker initiated these festivals, an attempt to bring the arts to people who wouldn't dream of crossing the threshold of a theatre or gallery. They're a quixotic attempt to prise culture free from the exclusions of class. When it works, it's moving.

In the Filton hangar, the sixteen-piece jazz band is unpacking its instruments, opening music stands. Lights flicker, people gather in knots. If enough come, the acoustic will be okay; if not, it could be muddy. They kick off with Take The A Train. *It works; the drive of piece is clear, the punchy riffs bite home, the solos soar. It's British jazz at its most confident, the music I've discovered at Ronnie Scott's, the sounds of Tubby Hayes, John Dankworth, Art Themen, British bebop, jazz dissolving cultural demarcations.*

People begin to dance. Standing by the bandstand, its stage manager for tonight, I watch young men and women jiving, whirling energetically, skirts flaring, mouths gaping, hearts racing, feet soft-shoe shuffling.

I see an exquisite creature spinning in the glitterball light. A slim sparrow of a woman, with blonde hair and honey-coloured skin. At the first opportunity I ask her to dance. She swings around me, I let her out, pull her in, the band's pumping, I'm in heaven.

This is how I meet Jane.

She asks me back to her place, halfway up the hill to Clifton. We spend the night together; the sun streams in next morning across our spent bodies. Her skin is like silk against mine, her hair strewn golden across the pillow.

More lovemaking, walking in the bright air along Clifton's white terraces, breathing deep. Few words, long looks into her grey-green eyes.

But I have to go back to London. I tear myself away and set out, promising I'll write from London –

– which I do, a tender letter, but with a piece of information I held back in Bristol. 'I'm engaged to be married next month,' I write. And then, in an impulse whose memory makes me shake my head in shame today, I ask her if she'll come to my wedding.

After a few days, Jane replies. She will come, with a mutual friend, Geoffrey, a whiz kid with lighting and projection. And she did, to the Grand Palais, Commercial Road, the last active Yiddish theatre in the East End, also available for weddings and barmitzvahs. *Arnold and Dusty Wesker did the catering, Geoffrey projected Buster Keaton movies on the walls, we danced to a quintet of players from the Big Band. Jane says hello by Geoffrey's side, smiling like a sphinx, inspecting Lis, now the first Mrs Kustow.*

Marriage moves in, I try to play the role of a devoted husband, and take my first steps into the theatre. I lose touch with Jane; I hear she's teaching in the East End. Her body dances in my memory.

We meet again, when I bring a touring group – an 'actors' commando' I called it – to the school where she's teaching. There's a flurry of emotion, my heart speeds up. But it's ships that pass: she's married by now.

My marriage goes downhill. I call Jane from Stratford upon Avon, where I'm working for the Royal Shakespeare Company, ask her to come and see me. It's a joyful, sexual, tearful reunion. But again, I can't seize her, I somehow don't feel I deserve her – and she's not even Jewish, which makes our love transgressive. So it's just a brief encounter, and we drift apart.

Years pass. We meet by chance, and begin our affair again. But now I'm running an arts centre, and tell myself I'm too wedded to work, I'm married to the ICA and have energy and Eros for little else. I remarry, to Orna, an Israeli. It goes well to begin with, then less well. One Sunday morning Jane greets me in the local greengrocer. I'm back from playing tennis. We go to the pub next door, which is festooned with bunting for the royal jubilee. We talk in broken sentences. She's been living four streets away. Now she has a daughter, but has left the daughter's father. We start up again. With the help of therapy and in the spirit of Woody Allen, I seriously consider leaving Orna for Jane. I walk round to Jane's flat. As I climb the stairs, my heart accelerates, again.

I leave home. I go back home, out of guilt and pity. This time it's going to be more than a brief encounter. I want to give and give. It's like being blinded by fierce white light which we, incandescent, give off.

Now, fourteen years later.

I finish writing an e-mail of pain to Jane, I feel calm. The grievous calm of depletion. I go to bed and sleep until 4am.

Jane comes down next morning, asks whether she should bring a newspaper back for me. She doesn't mention what I've written. I can't stand not knowing whether she has read it and has decided to ignore it or whether she hasn't, so I ask, 'Have you read your e-mails this morning?'

'Why?'

'Because I've written to you.'

'I thought you might,' she says.

She reads it, both my e-mail and a second one I added, quoting Louis Armstrong singing *Saint James Infirmary*, which was playing while I was writing: 'You may roam the wide world over / But you'll never find a lovin' man like me.'

There are tears in her eyes. I say nothing. I think for a second what a Bergmanesque scene this would make.

More silence. Jane looks from left to right, restlessly moving her head.

I ask her what she wants out of us.

'I don't know,' she says, through tears. 'I don't know what I want.'

That night I meet Kops at the Young Vic to see (in my case for a second time) Peter Brook's Beckett *Fragments*. Kops arrives in the theatre bar, a diminutive figure in a peaked cap – I suddenly see him, across the crowd of active young people using their cell phones and iPods, looking like a sailor from Holland, whence his family emigrated. I get out a book of Anthony Caro's sculptures of the gods and heroes of the Trojan War to show him; we've begun work on a screenplay which revolves around the theft of antiquities.

Across the road in a Turkish restaurant, I start talking about Jane, about her and me. He leaps at his thoughts, a habit which may be due to failing short-term memory (he's eighty-one) but is also his temperament, impulsive, immediate. 'You've got to see where she's coming from. She's angry, angry at the way your illness has hit her, and she can't help putting some of that anger onto you – "How could you do this to me?" She's irritated by some things you do, above all by your need to control. You are a *mensch*, Michael, but you have a need to control everyone and everything around you. Last week, in our class, I'd hardly got started before you challenged me.'

I protest that it's part of my nature – although I'm not so sure, I'm beginning to see it more as a reaction than an essence, a pre-emptive strike in my struggle with my father, grabbing the territory before he does so.

'No wonder you make Jane angry, and not just Jane. People feel your forcefulness, your need to take over. That's something I know in myself, but where you push out at people, I try to draw them in.'

A thought comes flooding back: when I split up with Lis, my first wife, she said, 'You trampled all over me.' I was astonished at the time, and for years later. Hadn't I always been an affectionate, loving husband? Now I glimpse the size of my narcissism, the need to assert and impose my ways of seeing, my sovereign self. It's a thought that haunts me through the evening, as Beckett's sad but utterly unsentimental clowns cavort before my eyes, circumnavigating the treadmill of life, the labyrinth of being lost like Dante in the dark wood. I have been domineering, shouldered my way into situations, but that's been inseparable from my activism and my prowess as a producer.

Kops saw this from the start, which is why we've become friends again so fast and why I relish him.

'Just look at you in the hospital ward – you weren't whimpering, Doctor, Doctor, am I going to be all right. You were like King Kustow, the bed your throne. You knew all the nurse's names, you were flirting with them, they loved it.'

I think he also sees the uncertainty, the wound, behind the ebullience which I've made my compensation. That's why he still thinks I qualify as being a *mensch*, a good-hearted person; I hope so anyway.

This also makes me think about my brother and my sister. He's been domineering in a different way, as a real estate developer. He cut the best deals, saw possibilities first, kept ahead of the pack. I've seen him acting larger than life in the office of his architect, playing to the gallery and believing that they love him for the glitz of it.

He's certainly a risk-taker, a gambler. I've also heard him humbled by the banks, when one of his gambles crashed. His drive stems from the same source as mine: fighting Dad, doing it differently from him, and better. In my brother's case, this was head-on defiance: he went out to play on the same pitch as his father, business. In my case, I sidestepped that confrontation, and went into a field where he couldn't compete: culture, learning, language. But the same rule of over-compensation applies, which may be why I became such a gobbler – of books, ideas, languages, and men and women. Now, late in the day, I'm trying to do more with less, and relish what and who I have, including my brother. Instead of accumulating, I'm trying to distil. This is one of the things this 'brush with death' has given me.

About my sister – no, it's much harder, it's too rich a soup, I don't know her so well, she's too far away in America. She's had two family hauntings to cope with: her mother's passivity as well as her father's panicky authoritarianism. She grew up in the culture of blame and, in this respect, mirrors our mother, a legacy she's trying to transcend.

I don't understand her grudge towards our brother. She's more or less given up on me, the brother who moved away from the family nexus, the knot that strangles.

All three of us siblings, second-generation English from a migrant family, have become over-reachers, each in his or her own way. This history also explains why I have such admiration for Pinter's *The Homecoming*, which, without being overtly and naturalistically Jewish, seems to me a universal archetype of the mechanisms of a family displaced, red in tooth and claw. A similar mythical story could be told of immigrant Irish, Caribbean, Indian, Bengali or Polish families. It's the situation, not the ethnicity, that's universal.

Watching Beckett's plays a second time, I notice how maniacally patterned his imagination is. These plays are permutations created by an obsessive/compulsive. In the novels it was the endless counting of the stones as they were transferred from one pocket to another;

in *Godot* it was permutations with shoes. Here, the antitheses and doublings become circus turns: in the first play, it's the interlocking of A, a blind beggar with B, a cripple in a wheelchair. In *Act Without Words II*, it's two antithetical men again: 'A is slow, awkward (dressing and undressing, gags), absent; B brisk, rapid, precise', says Beckett's stage direction. We watch them like circus spectators looking down into the ring as they work through the daily round of being prodded awake by a goad, praying, teeth-brushing, dressing, pulling along the sacks in which they've been sleeping, going to sleep again, being prodded awake again, praying...

But it's *Rockaby* that provides the most minimal glimpse into Beckett's twin-track mind. A woman alone, in a chair (Brook sacrifices a rocker; this is just a chair) speaking and rephrasing a mantra of loneliness, modifying it with minute changes, trying to edit it closer to the reality of her life. Until she is tipped out of it.

Kops watches entranced and troubled. 'It reminds me of when I was in the mental hospital in the 'fifties. It was full of obsessive people repeating their phrase with tiny alterations. Hour after hour. It's like minimal music: repetition with almost imperceptible changes.'

There are conkers underfoot. The air is warm and moist. This is a season of harvesting, not scattering seeds. Am I at last learning to do the same?

Friday, October 5, 2007

Tony Benn is waiting for us outside what we must now call 'Shakespeare's Globe', to distinguish it from a Shaftesbury Avenue competitor. Tonight this waterside Globe is giving the last performance of Jack Shepherd's play about the Chartists, *Holding Fire*, and we've invited Tony to join us. He accepted at once: 'We need the Chartists more than ever now.' Two hours before the performance, he phoned Jane and asked her if he might be permitted to say a few words from the stage at the end. I found the Globe's artistic director Dominic Dromgooole. He barely paused.

'Of course we'd like to have him. It would be an honour. But can he keep it short? Three minutes?'

Knowing Benn's platform precision and pithy concision, honed on countless rallies and debates and demonstrations, I say yes.

We're meeting him two years after he retired as an MP, to have, as he said, 'more time for politics', He's since worked as hard as ever, touring the country with a singer/songwriter in a solo show of political reminiscences and parables, becoming a figurehead of the anti-war movement and tirelessly taping his diaries, now totalling more than eighteen million words, and already a historical source.

This weekend he's particularly incensed, because the government has withdrawn its permission for Stop the War Coalition to demonstrate in Parliament Square next Monday, when Gordon Brown will be making a speech about Iraq in the Commons. A few days ago the police had stopped being helpful, and told the organisers they could not enter Parliament Square. Their authority was the 1839 law which had been used to stop the Chartists marching for universal suffrage. Benn has given notice that he and his fellow-marchers will not be deterred, in an open letter to the Home Secretary:

> I am writing to you as president of the Stop the War Coalition, to give you advance notice that there will be a demonstration in Trafalgar Square the day parliament meets calling for the immediate withdrawal of all British troops from Iraq and Afghanistan at which I shall be speaking along with others.
>
> Afterwards many of those present – including myself – will be marching along Whitehall to the House of Commons to meet MPs and urge them to support this call for a withdrawal, as I shall be doing in approaching Malcolm Rifkind my own local MP.

The authority for this march derives from our ancient right to free speech and assembly enshrined in our history, of which we often boast and which we vigorously defended in two world wars.

I climb up the Globe's wooden steps to our seats – benches without backs – a Spartan playhouse, built to be as accurate a copy as possible of Shakespeare's 'wooden O'. Tony Benn, in his well-weathered anorak, his extinguished pipe clutched in his hand, leans forward, eagerly gazing into the well of the theatre.

Mark Rosenblatt's production of Jack's play commandeers the entire space – thrust stage, galleries, yard for the promenading groundlings. Actors sweep in through the audience, leap up onto the stage, harangue each other above our heads. A Chartist leader is hanged from a scaffold erected among the groundlings; capital punishment at close-up range. The action pivots on two characters: Lovett, the gradualist, who believes that change can come cumula-tively, and O'Connor, the revolutionary who preaches violent action if necessary but is intimidated by a smooth-talking army captain and big green cannon, poking alarmingly from the stage. Through the story of these historical characters, Jack threads an imagined one, the story of a poor girl who joins the Chartists, whose lover is killed by the army, who will go on fighting, she says, for people's rights. A strong, simple story, the stuff of street ballads of the time.

Tony Benn nods approval of Lovett's closing speech: 'We're not asking for reform in the way that the beggar asks for a handout from his benefactors; what we demand is an equality of opportunity for every man, woman and child in this country.'

As the applause breaks out, I lead him through the crowd and up on stage, to even more applause. A slight, bright-eyed figure, he coasts and halts the clapping, thanks the performers, and gives us a crash course in radical politics, his family's connection with them, and the lesson that will still need to be enacted in two days' time on Whitehall and in Parliament Square. 'We need the two things the Chartists had,' he concludes. 'Anger and hope. Anger at the way things are, hope for the future.'

Theatre's truth-telling fictions spill over into the realities of a march, the power of many voices united under the skies. We leave elated. Tomorrow Tony will get up at dawn to join the postal workers on their picket line.

Chapter Seven:
CITY OF THE NEW

A Week in Paris, October 22–29, 2007

I walk from the Louvre through the Jardin des Tuileries to the Place de la Concorde and I realise why I feel so good in Paris. The spaces of the city set me up like a dancer. In Paris I cut a better shape in the air. The city observes me the way an audience observes a performer. I'm aware of façades behind me, perspectives stretching into the distance until they meet at some triumphal focal point; the Arc de Triomphe, the Bastille column, Sacré Coeur. A thousand mirrors reflect my body and its language. I am conscious of my outline, of the way I stand or strut. What a stage-set, what a décor Paris is! It frames you, feeds your dreams of yourself.

I carry with me a battered paperback of Ian Nairn's gazetteer of Paris, a clutch of brief love-letters to this creature, across whose body I pick my way.

> Nowhere else in Paris is the city's uniqueness presented with such conviction as in the Tuileries gardens. Because this end of the gardens is, simply, a gravelled space interrupted occasionally with grass and thickly planted with trees in a formal pattern. What's special about that? The scale and compassion of the gesture, which supplies basic amenity as though it were food and drink and then leaves you free – really free – to enjoy it.

Rhapsodically, Nairn nails my Paris – a well of experiences and discoveries, passions and illusions, of the new catching me by the throat and making my heart thump. This is my first trip abroad since the cancer, and I devour the sights and smells and tastes like a man set free – or at least out on reprieve. Women's impossibly long legs and determined strides. The ranks of patisseries in vitrines, the pyramids of fruit on parade – 'Don't touch *monsieur*, I will serve you.' Expansive hand gestures. Tender embraces in the middle of the pavement. The frank, appraising gaze I meet on the Metro, in lifts. Sexual promise.

Over the week, I stay with Marie-Thérèse in Pigalle, then in a small hotel in the Marais, aristocratic and Jewish. I eat Asiatic fast food alone; pasta with Jean-Luc, a bento lunch with Nina; fish with Marko and Marie-Hélène and oysters *fines claires* with Jacques and Nicole.

I look at Courbet's paintings – massive waves, languorous bodies, portraits of intelligent people, hunters and the hunted, an undercurrent of terror in his self-portrait. Soutine's thick brush-strokes churn me up, his red suffuses me. Steichen's photographs seduce me: twilit Manhattan, mannequins and actors, all of them white. He created *The Family of Man* exhibition I saw in the Festival Hall in London when I was sixteen, a horizon-opening post-war celebration of common humanity.

I shop: a red scarf for Jane, appliquéd with big flowers, a tweed cap for me, from an Anglophile shop on the boulevard des Capucines. And books, I can't resist the books: a catalogue about Jerry Siegel and Joe Schuster, the inventors of Superman, and other Jews in the comic-strip business. David Servan-Schreiber's *L'Anticancer*. A doctor who discovered he had brain cancer at the age of thirty-one, he's written a book which is partly a personal story but mostly a scientific account of things – diet, exercise and emotions – you can affect yourself which will combat cancer, or its return. I study Servan-Schreiber's pocket-sized diet guide which comes with the book, checking my own eating against it. Maybe this is shutting the door after the horse has bolted, but his book gives me pause.

I make plans to go to places, see films and plays – and then let the plans drop, stop in a café and sit and write. I sniff out my friendly cafes in each *quartier* like a dog looking for the right lamp-post.

Surprises happen. Walking back from the Bastille, I see a familiar small figure beating his way towards me, a Tibetan satchel over his shoulder, his hair upright in a permanent reflex of astonishment, like Tintin. It's another Peter – Peter Sellars, theatre-director, child-man, cultural agitator – whom I've known for twenty-five years, since Harvard, where he was an undergraduate and I was a member of the faculty.

'What are you doing here?' he asks.

'I'm on my way to see Peter Brook,' I say.

'I've just been to see him,' says Sellars. 'Are you coming to the screening of Mark Kidel's film tonight? It's about me. You're in it.'

I go to the screening, in a studio of L'Opéra de La Bastille, which is on strike. Kidel's film shows Sellars in full flood: joining a puppet troupe while still at school, then starting his own; at seventeen whisked off by his mother to Paris, where he saw plays directed by Roger Planchon and Patrice Chéreau and drank in classical music, jazz and painting; dynamiting student drama at Harvard with a *King Lear* set in an automobile graveyard and Handel's' *Orlando* re-set in present-day Cape Canaveral with the epic hero as an astronaut. Sellars' energy, his creative insolence, his crusading anger hit me again in these evoked productions, and all those which followed: Mozart/ Da Ponte operas updated to the US, in a diner on Cape Cod, a luxury apartment in New York's Trump Tower and Spanish Harlem; Sophocles' *Ajax* at the Kennedy Center in Washington, re-set in the Pentagon; Euripides' *The Children of Hecuba,* staged with a chorus of asylum-seekers and a post-performance debate about immigration; Handel's oratorio *Theodora* at Glyndebourne, ending with the slow death by phenol injection of the Christian martyrs, imprisoned in a brutal Guantánamo of steel trolleys and orange jump-suits.

Mark Kidel, a director with whom I worked at Channel 4, captures Sellars teaching at UCLA, bestriding a lecture-hall from podium to back row, lambasting his students like an elated preacher with exhortations to take nothing in America on trust, but to find their individual voices.

Afterwards, at the champagne reception, I hug Peter – he barely reaches my shoulder – and tell him, 'I've always thought of you as my double, my brother, my alter ego. If I'd have had a mother as supportive as yours, I might have… You're my might-have-been.'

He says, 'You shouldn't underestimate what you've done. There you were, out of the British establishment, keeping your foot in the door so that wild people like me could get in, get things made and shown. And you just kept on keeping that door open.'

Well, yes, Peter, and I'm touched. But now, late in the day I want to make my own things in my own voice, not just enable the talent of others.

Paris turns me into a astronaut, bouncing in slow motion through my memories. Fragments, memories, freed from gravity, float towards me.

Arriving in a hotel room in the Marais, we sink into the bed. Your eyes widen with excitement. The day outside is bright, the light streams in, we have no deadlines, no occupations, no roles, your arms are long and smooth, your legs opening. You await me, as the city does. Afterwards, my knees are easy, my lungs open, my heart calm. Emptying into you, I feel clear, and a new day beckons.

Guillaume Apollinaire, poet of yearning, master of eroticism, shrapnel-pierced World War One soldier, caught this plenitude after sex, as he caught the cresting wave of desire before it, in the never-ending river of time.

Sous le pont Mirabeau coule la Seine
Et nos amours
Faut-il qu'il m'en souvienne
La joie venait toujours après la peine

Richard Wilbur translates this as

Under the Mirabeau bridge there flows the Seine
Must I recall
Our loves recall how then
After each sorrow joy came back again

In 1968 I co-wrote a play with Adrian Henri about Apollinaire, and staged it in the little theatre we'd carved out of the ICA gallery. It was called *I Wonder,* our translation of Apollinaire's *J'Emerveille* – 'I marvel at', but we liked the several meanings of *I Wonder*: 'I muse on this world and my place in it'; 'I am a wonder myself'. A wolfish-looking actor called Tom Kempinski played Apollinaire; a blonde actress the woman he worshipped; a slinky black actress the many more women he bedded. We conjured up his life *et ses amours* on the Somme battlefields, his astonishment at the spectacular fireworks of war, his insistence on seeing it as a carnival, a cavalcade – *Dieu, que La Guerre Est Jolie!*

Apollinaire opened the door for me to modernism, of which Paris remains the capital. He set French poetry free from its metrics in his own classical and colloquial poems, his *calligrammes* setting out words as patterns, as pictures, so rainfall became slanting lines of monosyllables down the page. His poems were as immediate as graffiti, they sang. After him came all the poets of the natural speaking voice, Louis Aragon, Blaise Cendrars, Paul Éluard, Jacques Prévert, Neruda, Cavafy, Ferlinghetti, suppressing punctuation and hanging on line-endings, poised at a summit before tumbling into bed with the next line.

Through Apollinaire's eyes I looked at Picasso and Braque's 1912 Cubist collages, their splintered perspectives, paint and cardboard becoming sculpture. Paris revealed the tightrope-walkers of modern art and sent me running after them, after Satie and Stravinsky, a very Parisian Russian; after Corbusier's cradling shapes; through to the improvisatory wit of Godard, his citations of book titles and phrases turning the screen into a page, his Apollinaire-esque *amour fou* for Anna Karina.

This was, this remains, my Paris: a shower for all the senses, a vortex of the new, capital of pleasure and of pain.

How many times I walked moodily along *quais* and *boulevards*, a solitary wanderer, and watched the sun come up across cupolas and squares, the moon reflected in the rippling river, cherishing love and the pang of its passing. *L'amour s'en va comme cette eau courante*: All love goes by as water to the sea / All love goes by.

London is a metropolis, a carpet of changing moods, monuments and markets, the lofty and the down-to-earth. Apollinaire stood on the Pont Mirabeau; Wordsworth, a century earlier, on Westminster Bridge reflected not on love passing but on the beauty of a busy city about to wake up:

> Shops, towers, domes, theatres and temples lie
> Open unto the fields, and to the sky
> All bright and glistening in the smokeless air.

Pre-industrial London, a place of business and trade for the English poet; for the French one, pre-First World War Paris a capital of romanticism. I inhabit both.

The other passion I learned from Paris – and indeed from my earlier year in Villeurbanne – was political passion.

One day in autumn 1961, after a night in a cheap hotel in Lyon, I made my way to the main square of its suburb Villeurbanne, the Place Lazare-Goujon. There, between the police station and the municipal swimming pool, was my destination, a theatre, Le Théâtre de la Cité. I'd come from Israel, where a three-month stint on a kibbutz in Galilee had left me healthy, indoctrinated with Zionism and missing Europe. I was carrying a sack of unresolved Jewishness on my English back. But after three months I was no nearer solving the dilemma of being a Jew in England, belonging and not belonging, weighing allegiances.

Besides, I'd left a girlfriend behind in Oxford; more unfinished business. I decided I had to get back and see her, and rang her from Villeurbanne to say I was returning.

'Don't,' she said. 'We agreed to separate for a year and then see.'

So I decided to stay in France, and to see the work of this theatre. I turned up next day and asked if I could join the theatre.

'Why not?' said their General Manager, Jean-Marie Boeglin. 'Come to rehearsals, watch, learn, we can't pay you; maybe you can find a job teaching English. Come back tomorrow and I'll take you into rehearsals.'

Next day I asked for Monsieur Boeglin.

'Haven't you read your papers?' they said, 'Jean-Marie won't be here. He's fled to Switzerland.'

Boeglin, I learned, had been part of a *réseau de soutien*, a support network for the Algerian nationalists, the *Front de Liberation Nationale* (FLN), fighting for independence from France since 1958, raising money, smuggling weapons. They were marked men; the police had decided to swoop. Some were caught; others, like Boeglin, got away, became political exiles.

I went to court to follow the trial of the *réseau* members. There were seven of them: five Algerians and two Frenchmen. They were led into court in chains, and given jail sentences. The sound of those clanking chains haunted me.

Over the next year, as I taught English at the École Berlitz, went to rehearsals, was taken on by the theatre, wore seventeenth-century costume and waved banners and danced the cha-cha in *Les*

Trois Mousquetaires, the conflicts in France got worse. The *Organisation Armée Secrète* (OAS), a far-right militant outfit, planted bombs outside left-wingers' apartments and in cafés and cinemas. The FLN retaliated with its own acts of terrorism in mainland France. A curfew was imposed. Thirty thousand Algerians marched against it in Paris. They met a massive police force. Demonstrators were beaten, shot, drowned in the Seine.

Georges Wilson's *Théâtre National Populaire* put on a season of anti-war and anti-fascist plays: Brecht's *Arturo Ui* and Aristophanes' comedy *Peace*, adapted by Sartre. The corridors of the theatre at the Palais de Chaillot rang with laughter and rage.

Rumours began that a bunch of disaffected generals, convinced that de Gaulle had betrayed them, were preparing a *putsch*, a takeover to install a junta. On April 23 1961, Shakespeare's birthday, I was in a coach with my French theatre friends speeding towards our next tour date, in Stuttgart. The radio in the coach was saying that the *putschistes* had half the army and the air force behind them; the *putsch* would begin with a massive parachute drop on Paris and other major cities, and citizens were urged to go to the airports and resist the plotters.

It was pouring that day. On the other lane of the *Autobahn* we could see grey-green columns of tanks and armoured trucks heading from their German NATO bases towards Paris. Panic took hold in the coach. Our families are at risk, said some. But maybe the French soldiers are going to Paris to support de Gaulle, said others.

We entered Stuttgart at dusk. Some actors wanted to go straight to their hotel rooms. Wait, said others, de Gaulle is about to broadcast. The booming voice of the old man began: *'Françaises, Français...'*

The plotters wavered; de Gaulle won. (Seven years later he was to outface the students and workers of the 1968 *évènements* with similar theatrical skill.) In 1962, he granted Algeria its independence. Within a year, Algerian nationalists had split into factions. Heroes of the Resistance were damned as enemies of the state. I wondered what had happened to Jean-Marie Boeglin, who had emigrated and thrown in his lot with the Algerian revolution.

I was living through events a world away from the black and white righteousness of the Campaign for Nuclear Disarmament, which had given me my first experience of a political movement. The Algerian war and its aftermath was my political baptism of fire, my first taste of political struggle and defeat, of the way political idealism and solidarity could give rise to recriminations and splits.

I go to see Peter Brook in his loft near the Bastille. He opens the door, takes me by the shoulders and gives me a long gaze from those searching, stone-grey eyes. 'I hear from many sources that there's a new serenity about you, Michael,' he says.

The loft has been repainted since I last came. A baby grand piano, given to Peter by his parents, stands at the far end. There are fewer books, less things altogether. On a long shelf, he's placed six little statues. An owl, which I take to be Athena's owl of wisdom, but which turns out to be the work of Peter's son Simon, made when he was at school. Several Pre-Columbian figures. Two little icons, paintings, one of Saint George killing a spiky dragon, the other, Peter says, given to him by an old icon-painter in Jerusalem who recognised in Peter a kindred spirit.

We sit in upright chairs on an oriental carpet, two feet apart. We talk about his plans and travels – he's off to Morocco next day, to work with a group on 'some Gurdjieff material'. Next year he will take a group of actors to Israel and Palestine, to workshop *Eleven and Twelve*, a play about a Sufi peacemaker in a West African Muslim community split apart by a disagreement over whether a certain prayer should be recited eleven or twelve times in the daily litany.

This play is Peter's testimony, perhaps: a fable about the power and fragility of 'right action', a searing picture of chauvinism and colonial rule, an example of his cross-culturalism, especially his love of the exuberance and stillness of African actors. Having done it in

French, he's revised it and will do it in English, this time adding Palestinian actors to the cast. In Israel and the West Bank, he plans to rehearse, take episodes of the piece out into villages and schools, and open it in Ramallah and Jerusalem. Theatre crossing political borders, speaking in its own voice across the political babble.

During my illness, he's been a real friend, calling me in the hospital almost daily from wherever he was touring. Writing his biography might have meant the end of our friendship, as many biographers of living people have found. But it hasn't.

Peter's brother Alexis, a distinguished psychotherapist, died three months ago. The two brothers had an affectionate closeness, which Simon, Peter's son, captured in his documentary about his father, *Brook by Brook*. At the funeral service in Golders Green Crematorium, among a flock of psychotherapists from the Tavistock Clinic, Peter spoke with the simplicity of a son and a brother. It's as if he's shedding his brilliance and conquistador energy as he grows older, to make way for a simpler stillness, a less demonstrative way of being in the world.

He talks about 'the invisible face of things'; is other-worldly and at the same time very deeply of this world. I'm aware of the well of what I can only call belief from which he draws, but he's also living a full life of the body and the mind in the here and now.

I imagine him submitting to the authority of his group, perhaps one of the few times he does so in a life of mastery and conquest. He confronts the major perceptions of Gurdjieff, Grotowski, the *Bhagavad Gita* and The Grand Inquisitor.

Living between French and English gives him a scalpel-like edge. English provides more jokes. He writes with crisp French concision and balance.

Meetings with Remarkable Men is his most personal film, and the most independent of all genres and styles. His Gurdjieff connection is confidential, and I am wary of the loose language of 'spirituality' when I ask about this part of him. There's a rigour and sharpness in his words when he speaks of it. What I am sure of is that, had he not discovered Gurdjieff as a young man, his talent and appetite and hunger for life would have swamped him. He learned a way to channel these things, a map of his energy, with experiences in proportion and connection to each other. This is a lesson I am still learning.

When I ask him a question, there's often a long pause before he replies; the cog-wheels of his mind rapidly revolving all the facets of possible answers. Usually, he starts his reply from a distant and unexpected corner.

He's drawn to the mystery of the mind. Oliver Sacks' *The Man who Mistook his Wife for a Hat*. Alexander Luria's *The Mind of a Mnemonist*. He made shows of them both. Can science lead him to a human essence? Is there a theatrical image that can gather up philosophy, theory and clinical practice? He loves actors, they are his material, anchoring speculation. He's looking for acting that is not confined by cultural borders; all this long before 'multi-culturalism'.

He's drawn to peacemakers, like Tierno Bokar, the strength of the powerless. He could be the abbot of a Zen monastery, or a Sufi sage. He is a connoisseur of paradox, a devotee of freedom, moved by the struggles of the South African townships, and the wry zest of black South African actors. His stillness, his capacity to wait, are lessons to me.

Thursday, November 8, 2007

A witness says that when he opened the doors of the gas chamber, there were bodies holding fistfuls of hair. Another witness remembers corpses with flesh sliced off their bones, women with their breasts cut off. Another, asked by the prosecutor to identify a defendant, points to a man in the second row of the audience at the Young Vic.

This is Peter Weiss' *The Investigation*, performed by seven actors from a Rwandan company. They move calmly, speak their French text carefully, never lose touch with us. 'We survived the camps, but the camps are still with us.' They wear white and cream-coloured suits, take off their jackets and put them on again, move into new groupings. Each of them plays both victim and persecutor. Twice, they sing: snatches of a rich, close-harmonised African song. They make a sculptural group. Like Rodin's *Burghers of Calais*, who sacrificed themselves to save their besieged city, they stand powerless before us, lit from above, then below, then from side to side. Their succession of horrendous stories morph into a surreal nowhere and everywhere, an unending nightmare which is taking place in a Nazi camp in 1944, in Rwanda fifty years later. And in Darfur now.

I take my head in my hands, and I notice that I am breathing deeply in order not to close myself to it, to take every detail in.

I've read a handful of books about the death-camps – Hilberg, Gilbert, Davidowicz – but by and large have kept away from the Holocaust. It's too much exploited by some of my fellow Jews to justify Israel's actions today. But seeing this piece in the shared space of the Young Vic, the stage and the audience in a single room, makes it mandatory to remember. In 1965, when I was at the Royal Shakespeare Company, Peter Brook and David Jones staged a reading of Weiss's 'oratorio-stage-documentary' late at night in the Aldwych Theatre, simultaneously with thirteen theatres in East and West Germany. 'With more time,' wrote Brook, 'we could have prepared a more polished performance, built a set, made music. What for? We feel our job is to transmit this text at once – to whom it may concern.' At the Young Vic now, the Rwandan company hold up the conflicting accusations, lies and excuses in a web of beauty. But because of the experience of their country, there's nothing aestheticising about it; it's an urgent cry of alarm.

Seeing *The Investigation* fits into a cluster of other experiences. I'm reading a book about Theodore Herzl, the founder of Zionism, who in 1896 in *The State of the Jews* uncannily predicted the 'clash of civilisations' theory of today: 'For Europe, we shall serve there as part of the fortified wall against Asia, and function as the vanguard of civilisation against the Barbarians.' In three weeks, I go to Israel and Palestine for ten days.

At the Young Vic people stand and cheer the cast. That seems wrong. I know it's a way of showing solidarity with the actors, but maybe silence would be better. We walk out of the theatre. I don't feel like just taking the Tube and going home by myself. Jane is in Southampton, giving a talk about Afghanistan to a Stop the War group – 'Probably ten people and a dog,' she says, before setting out. 'It's your commitment,' I say. 'But maybe Stop the War has passed its peak.' 'Not if Iran is attacked,' she says.

I decide to get off the train at St Pancras and take a look at the new rail terminal, which will bring Europe, via Eurostar, closer to where I live. Gilbert Scott's Gothic palace adjoining the station, soon to become a luxury hotel (run by The Manhattan Loft Company, says the billboard) is lit with a battery of spotlights washing the red brick walls, and columns of orange light picking out its verticals.

The entrance to the station is barred by security men: some VIP event is in progress. 'Who are the fat cats tonight?' I ask a black security man. 'Travel agents,' he says.

I know I will fall in love with the new St Pancras, its atrium of humanity on the move. I know my heart will lift the way it does when I visit Grand Central Station – or the lofty entrance hall of University College Hospital. Arrivals and departures, entrances and exits, people seeking directions – which do I love more, hospitals or railway stations?

Next week is Blake's two hundred and fiftieth birthday, and there's a host of events to mark the day. I won't be in London, but flying to the place that so inspired Blake, Jerusalem. I rejoice, not just in Blake's

And we shall build Jerusalem
In England's green and pleasant land

which has stirred English radicals and revolutionaries, but in his
poetic vision of London, seeing Jerusalem peeping through its
streets:

The fields from Islington to Marylebone
To Primrose Hill and Saint John's Wood
Were builded over with pillars of gold
And there Jerusalem's pillars stood

Her Little-ones ran on the fields
The Lamb of God among them seen
And fair Jerusalem his Bride
Among the little meadows green

Pancras and Kentish Town repose
Among her golden pillars high
Among her golden arches which
Shine upon the starry sky

I've been thinking about Chaim Soutine again today, an aftershock
of seeing fifty Soutine paintings in Paris last month. His red punched
into my body.

Red of flushed cheeks
Red of a soubrette's hair
Red for the page-boy's uniform
Red in a swirl of space
    Yellow blue black
Red of the poppy
    In the buttonhole of the crumpled shirt

Red against the black
    Of Soutine's sad defiant eyes

Red for the sides of beef
    In his butcher block pictures
    Next to silver of fish on plates

Red like the tip of my stoma
    Poking through the hole in my belly

Chapter Eight:
THE PUNISHED LAND

Israel / Palestine, November 2007

I come to Tel Aviv, to see friends and theatre, and to go to Hebron and Jenin to see the occupied West Bank. This must be at least my twentieth trip to Israel since 1959, when I came on a Jewish Agency tour at the end of my first year at Oxford and returned home to write an elated article for the student newspaper. It was inspired by the idea of battered and almost extinguished Jews putting themselves together in Zionist/Tolstoyan kibbutzim. The illustrations – photographs of Zionist maidens picking apples – were courtesy of the Jewish Agency.

Two years later, I went to a kibbutz, where I picked apples, collected garbage and did not find the elusive Grail that might have made sense of my Anglo-Jewishness. I could have given Israel more of a chance – lived in Tel Aviv or Jerusalem, met kindred spirits, done a master's degree in Kafkaology or something. But I missed Europe, came back, put Israel on the back burner, until I met and married Orna from Haifa. After that, I came to Israel at least once a year, to meet my in-laws and her friends, and make my own. Then we divorced, and Israel moved out of the foreground. Now I am critical of Israel's policies while loving the place and probably knowing more Israelis closely than many other critics in England.

Rina

I have dinner with Rina Yerushalmi, Israel's best theatre director and, together with Pina Bausch and Ariane Mnouchkine, one of the outstanding women directors in the world. It's Friday night, so not much is open, and we choose Keton, on Dizengoff, which serves the kind of food my grandmothers might have cooked – boiled chicken with *tsimmes*, a comforting mush of sweet potatoes and prunes, followed by strudel. In her sixties, Rina has cropped hair, a penetrating mind and a slightly melancholic air, but a hearty laugh. She began as a dancer, and became a pupil of Moshe Feldenkrais, a remarkable Russian-born movement teacher, formerly a Judo Black Belt and physicist. He gave Rina a deep grounding in his method, and her version of it underpins the troupe of young actors she leads.

What really bowled me over four years ago was her two-evening staging of the central stories of the Old Testament, *Vayomer Vayelech* (And he Spoke, and he Went), which she patiently built up over four years.

We sat on three sides of a big rehearsal room backstage at the Cameri Theatre. Light sculpted the space; music conjured up tribal rage and excitement; sounds of wind and rain opened perspectives of distance and desert. A dozen young actors, clad in elegant black, moved slowly in. I had heard many of them speaking Shakespeare in Hebrew translation, but the text of their Bible, reeling out waves of ancestors, lists of prohibitions, battle strategies and sexual interdictions, offered them a new intimacy and confidence with their language.

But there was nothing antiquarian about Rina's production. We might have been watching a chic group of nightclubbers, starting a Biblical cabaret. All the Hebrew Bible's greatest hits were there, Adam and Eve in the Garden of Eden were refracted into a chorus of couples, the women proffering the apple of pleasure and sin, the men attacking the apples with knives and forks. The Ten

Commandments, thundered out by a hellfire preacher, material-
ised as comic-strip tableaux. The Golden Calf was danced/spoken
by an Amazonian actress wearing an animal skull on her head; an
elemental apparition.

When the Flood hit the wicked children of Israel, it killed them in
paroxysms of writhing, gasping helplessness – an image, it seemed, of
Israeli fears of Saddam's Scud missiles only a few years before, when
families had shut themselves into air-proof shelters. When the tribes
of Israel went out as exiles, they carried the battered suitcases of
refugees of all ages. And when their sons were called up for military
service to fight the enemy, it tapped into every family's apprehen-
sions about war. Rina's Bible show re-imagined King David as a
red-nosed clown, and Biblical legislators as the forerunners of every
bent-backed regulator. It was mythical theatre rooted in the body,
speaking not only to Jews, but to every diasporic people, trudging
from one stopover to the next with their valises and bundles, in
search of The Promised Land.

Shaike

From the 1960s until five years ago when he died, Shaike Weinberg
was one of my main reasons for coming to Israel. Shaike (a diminutive of 'Isaiah' in Hebrew) became something between a hero and a
father-figure for me.

'I am Weimar,' Shaike told me, 'a little adulterated by the Middle
East.' He told me I didn't have to struggle so hard to make sense of
being Jewish. 'You are a Jew whatever you do.'

When I saw him for the last time in 2000, he was sitting in his
flat in Jabotinsky Square with a glass of Scotch, reading Daniel
Singer's *Whose Millennium?*, a last-testament summation of the
legacy of socialism and a philippic against the inevitability of capi-
talism. Singer, like Shaike, a Polish Jewish socialist in the tradition of

Rosa Luxemburg, outlines a post-millennial society, international-ist, egalitarian and truly democratic. As we entered his room, Shaike shut the book with impatience. 'I can see the destination,' he said. 'But where's the agency?'

We're still looking for it.

Born in Warsaw, educated in Weimar Berlin, Shaike carried into the culture of Israel the questioning and cosmopolitan socialism which was one of the best legacies of the emancipation of the Jews in Europe. Whether running a challenging theatre or creating a succession of pioneering museums, his principled inventiveness kept everyone around him honest.

Berlin sharpened his wit and shaped his politics. When Jane and I went to see him in Tel Aviv not long before his death, he proudly showed us his father's library of first editions of Marx, Lassalle and other Marxist classics – and a collected Heine. He was annoyed that he couldn't lay his hands on his Rosa Luxemburg volumes.

In 1935, he and his family emigrated to Palestine. For twenty years he worked on a left-wing kibbutz. He fought against British rule in the Hagana, then in 1942 became a British army sergeant in the Jewish Brigade. He led his troops – many of whom had lost families in the death camps – from Italy up to the Austrian border. With the help of British intelligence, accounts were settled with known Nazi killers. Today we would call it targeted assassination, conducted by the relatives of the victims.

Shaike set up the Israeli government's first mainframe computer, in the office of the prime minister. Four years later he was asked by a group of talented actors, who he had met in the British Army, to run Tel Aviv's Cameri Theatre, which they were forming as a modern alternative to the Habimah theatre.

For sixteen years he ran the Cameri, in the mould of Brecht's Berliner Ensemble and Jean Vilar's Théâtre National Populaire. As a giddy triumphalism succeeded the victories of the 1967 Six-Day War, Shaike staged Hanoch Levin's caustic satires, despite political pressure from the Cameri board, which included Leah Rabin, wife of the future prime minister.

While running the theatre, he was asked to strike out in an entirely new direction. Nahum Goldmann, the independent-minded President of the World Jewish Congress, another product of the conjunction of Jews and German-language culture, convinced Shaike that one of Israel's greatest needs was a dynamic museum of the Diaspora. The younger generation had short memories, and tended to see Jewish life before the creation of the state of Israel as negligible and incomplete.

With Goldmann's diplomatic and financial backing, Shaike devised a radical museum, *Beth Hatefutsoth* (The House of the Diaspora), on the Tel Aviv University campus. Most historical museums, he argued, were built around the artefacts they happened to possess. But he intended to put historical narrative before objects, to exhibit facsimiles of lost Jewish objects made by craftsmen from the best surviving evidence. He yoked Disneyland techniques to serious historical scholarship.

The pre-eminence of this work in Tel Aviv led Shaike to be head-hunted as the founding director of the United States Holocaust Memorial Museum in Washington. Moving in when the project had begun, but had not yet found its way, Shaike's dialectical mind saw that the only way forward was to embody the inevitable tensions of its subject.

The museum should bring to life the historical narrative of an unequalled slaughter, but not become an exclusive memorial. Leading an international team of scholars, architects and designers, involving Holocaust survivors in selecting exhibits, dealing with the personalities of private donors and the demands of the US government (the museum had been granted a site near the Vietnam war memorial), Shaike deployed his talents.

It was often harrowing work. Shaike chaired the committee which decided whether to accept gifts of objects for the permanent display.

At one meeting they were confronted with a heap of human hair. 'We cannot have this,' said one survivor. 'My mother's hair might be in there.'

As a theatre-maker, Shaike valued plot, narrative and design. It was the plot, rooted in authoritative scholarship and realised in a spatial *mise en scène,* that squeezed maximum meaning out of the artefacts of mass killing. An Auschwitz cattle-truck, through which you were obliged to walk, tiny white figures of prisoners and guards in a miniature crematorium, resting on a case of Zyklon B canisters. A heap of dead Jews' worn shoes, stinking under the display lights. A battered milk-churn from the Warsaw ghetto, in which a fighter had stuffed his diary, hoping that it would be read by generations after his death.

> Turning the corner in the museum
> On your left you come across
> A battered milk-churn
>
> Emmanuel Ringelblum, memorialist,
> Buried it the day before the annihilation
> Of the Warsaw ghetto
>
> Milk-churn of memory:
> Diaries, documents, decrees, posters
> Maps of the camps
>
> Underground newspapers
> Concert tickets, milk coupons, chocolate wrappers
> A narrative of the deportations
>
> Burnished by spotlight
> Encrusted with clay
> It is as golden as the mask of Agamemnon
> The helmet of Achilles
> A capsule of mementoes
> On spaceship earth

Seven Role-Plays for the Occupation

To read on this trip I have brought with me Eyal Weizman's magisterial *Hollow Land: Israel's Architecture of Occupation*. I imagine myself a theatre director, leading a class of 'role-plays' for occupiers.

1.

You are a member of the Israeli army and have to pacify a Palestinian refugee camp. You know such camps are the 'hotbeds' of your enemies. They know you are coming, and have already blocked the main roads into the camp. Although you could smash through their barriers, you know they will hit you with merciless sniper fire. You have to flush them out, without using the roads and alleys of the camp. You have to go into people's homes.

This is what you do, as described by Eyal Weizman and his interviewees.

You position your squad outside the house wall. Military intelligence will have already given you a computer model of the house – every Palestinian house in Gaza and the West Bank has been mapped digitally in three dimensions. Using explosives or a large hammer, you punch a hole through the wall and climb in shouting. It is important to shout. You may throw in a stun grenade before entering the living room.

Aisha, a young Palestinian woman, describes what it feels like if you are an inhabitant.

> You're sitting in your living room, where the family watches television after the evening meal… The wall disappears with a deafening roar, the room fills with dust and debris, and through the wall pours one soldier after another, screaming orders. You have no idea if they're after you, if they've come to take over your home or if your home just lies on the route to somewhere else. The children are screaming, panicking. Is it possible even

to imagine the horror experienced by a five-year-old child as four, six, eight, twelve soldiers, their faces painted black, submachine guns pointed everywhere, antennas protruding from their backpacks, making them look like giant alien bugs, blast their way through the wall.

[All witnesses quoted come from Weizman's interviews]

2.

This is what you do if you are an Israeli town-planner intending to grab Palestinian land. You invent a new, constantly shifting legal terminology, masking your aims with sanitised words like 'survey land', 'state land', 'security land', all of which enable your nation to seize the land without recourse. You know that most Palestinians are too poor or intimidated to go to court to contest your actions. You dig out a land law of 1858 from the Ottoman Empire. It provides that if a farmer has not cultivated his land for three consecutive years, he forfeits ownership. Since you have cut off his water, he has not been able to farm the land, so Bob's your uncle, another tract of earth to add to the Land of Israel.

3.

If you are a judge in Israel's High Court of Justice, this is what you do. You know that your government has accepted Hague regulations and conventions defining the rights of civilians and the duties of armed forces in situations of 'belligerent occupation'. Under these principles, land may only be requisitioned in case of 'urgent military necessity' or 'benefit to the local population'. Even then, the takeover of the land is only 'temporary.'

When Palestinians and Israeli human rights groups petition the High Court against such requisitions, you reject them because, in the words of Justice Vitkon in 1978,

There can be no doubt that the presence...of settlements – even 'civilian' ones – of the administering power makes a significant contribution to the security situation in that territory and facilitates the army's performance of its tasks... These are simple matters and there is no need to elaborate.

4.

This is what you do if you are a Palestinian policeman on duty at a frontier checkpoint, regulating the movements of Palestinians. Sitting in front of a mirror, you take the applicant's passport, examine it, put it into a drawer beneath your desktop. Behind you, an Israeli security official takes the passport, runs it through computer checks and returns it with either a red label permitting the owner to enter or a white label refusing them permission to do so.

This is what is known as 'Palestinian autonomy'.

The mirror is one-way, like the policy that erected it.

At another checkpoint, the turnstile entrances have been narrowed, the better to detect metal weapons or bombs tied to the body. People who are wider than the opening get stuck. A bottle-neck results. It is very hot in the entrance tunnel of the checkpoints.

If you are an Israeli soldier on duty at a checkpoint, you may simply decide to shut up shop for an hour, several hours, even a day. It's completely random, like the cases reported by the women's organisation *Machsom* [Checkpoint] *Watch* of soldiers detaining every ninth man, or everyone called Mohammad. Little games to ease boredom. It gets stifling in the queue. The drinks and fast-food stalls which have gathered round the checkpoints do a roaring trade, one of the few flourishing sectors of the stricken Palestinian economy.

5.

This what you write if you are against what your government is doing:

Temporariness is now the law of the occupation...temporary encirclement and temporary closures, temporary transit permits, temporary revocation of transit permits, temporary enforcement of an elimination policy, temporary change in the open-fire orders... The occupier is an unrestrained, almost boundless sovereign, because when everything is temporary almost anything, any crime, any form of violence is acceptable, because the temporariness grants it a license, the license of the state of emergency.

You find yourself describing an Alice-through-the-Looking-Glass world, where everything is topsy-turvy, where a dozen different 'master plans' from competing generals or politicians, or generals hoping to become politicians, may disagree on details but all lead to the same destination: dispossessions of Palestinians. Eyal Weizman in his book calls this state of things 'an Escher painting'. In the work of that hallucinatory Dutch graphic artist, the foreground suddenly becomes the background, black becomes white, concave becomes convex and temporary means forever. So it goes in Gaza and the West Bank.

6.

Eyal Weizman, a young Tel Aviv architect opposed to the occupation, decided to fight it with his professional skills. Working with the human rights organisation B'tselem, taking aerial photographs of the Territories, digging into municipal records and obliging the Israeli government to make public its master-plans for settlement expansion and land annexation, he made a new map. It showed the location and extent of every settlement, extended city limit and military base in Israel and its occupied land. It charts every encroachment. It looks like a diseased lung.

This map is the basis of *Hollow Land*, Weizman's calmly devastating account of the bent laws and shifting regulations, the tactically vague language, the rivalries between power-hungry generals and the sheer *chutzpah* which has enabled Israeli planners and regulators to get away with the takeover. As a Jew I am ashamed to see such ingenuity and energy, such high-tech jargon and theory poured into ever-more inventive ways of, forgive the expression, fucking up the neighbour. Is this what the spirit of Maimonides, Spinoza and Heine has engendered? Have the theologians, the philosophers, the poets given birth to a new wave of academicians of counter-insurgency, inverting the subversive insights of Foucault and Deleuze not to demystify power but to mask it. Does the work of the military analysts of Zion provide a test-bed for America's 'war against terror'?

7.

This is what happened to Eyal Weizman. In 2002 he and his partner Rafi Segal won a competition to design the Israeli pavilion at the World Congress of Architecture in Berlin. The content of their pavilion, they announced, would be an exhibition called *The Politics of Israeli Architecture*. Drawing on Eyal's maps and researches, it would be the first international display of the spatial form of the settlements and the political and military policies that underpin the settlers' ranch houses and gardens and swimming pools on the West Bank hilltops, safe and comfortable 'gated communities' like those of South Africa or California.

Shortly before the congress, the invitation to Weizman and Segal was withdrawn by the Israeli Association of United Architects, and they were forbidden to distribute their catalogue. The association's head said,

> The association thinks that the ideas in the catalogue are not architecture. Heaven help us if this is what Israel has to show. As though only settlements...were built here... My natural

instincts tell me to destroy the catalogues, but I won't do that. I won't burn books.

Schwebel

We go to see Schwebel, high in the hills of Judea above the village where John the Baptist is supposed to have been born. Born in West Virginia seventy-five years ago, and growing up in the Bronx, Schwebel arrived in Jerusalem in 1963, after being in the US Army in Japan. There he'd found a Kyoto Zen master of drawing, who taught him the power of black, grey and white. Back in New York, he studied art history and went to art classes under Philip Guston. His marriage broke up, he went to Paris, tried to settle in Spain, but his money ran out.

'One girl after the other,' he says to me, 'led me to an empty house in the hills of Judea, which immediately I recognised, as a native Bronx boy, as paradise! No electricity, who needs electricity? No water, we'll get water from some place!'

He squatted in the old stone house, which he later bought, built on a studio and a couple of outhouses which wouldn't look out of place in an allotment.

Schwebel a man of cities, looks like a *kibbutznik* with his baseball-player's physique, shorts and digger's boots. I first met him thirty years ago walking in the hills above Ein Karem; I saw this figure stripped to the waist working with a sledge-hammer on the hillside, repairing the terraces. Sinatra was playing on a ghetto-blaster. He offered me a whisky, and we wound up drunkenly singing show-stopping numbers from American musicals.

'I asked myself, What is this big thing about Jerusalem?' he says. 'Somebody said: read the book of Samuel, read it, you're in David's city, read it! And of course I had never read it, so I read it, with a little help from friends, and I realised what it was all about! The energy that came out of the Book of Samuel is very real, the history was biting, the politics dirty and the love as strong and the killing as bloody as you could make it. I liked that, I said Well this is us, this reflects us!'

Schwebel's paintings and engravings, diaries and artist's books centred around King David, are set in the streets of today's Jerusalem and up in its hills. Realist painting meets abstraction in a blaze of fierce colours and photographic precision, shadowed by Israel's history. 'With the war in Lebanon I began to take this thing seriously. I found a parallel between what went on in the internal politics of this country, the struggle between left and right, the invasion of Lebanon, and what took place in the Book of Samuel. This overlapping caught me and I went with it.'

Schwebel's later series of David paintings are darker, full of David's vulnerability, mirroring Israel's inner nightmare that force alone cannot solve everything. His hero's narrative began to be punctuated by images of Israelis huddling in gas masks against Saddam's Scud missiles. He dragged his David into a Nazi death camp, subjecting his Old Testament power to the ultimate assault on Jews. He painted him in slurring strokes, smashed by the bullet of Yitzhak Rabin's assassin.

We sit in his kitchen, over a bottle of red wine from the Golan Heights. He's meeting Jane for the first time, and, like every Israeli friend who met her for the first time on this trip, he's impressed, not only by her beauty but by the precision of her questions and criticisms, and by the romantic story of how we re-met after decades and got together; a story which Jane hones with each telling.

Getting her to come to Israel at all has been a struggle; she imagined having non-stop arguments with Israelis. That hasn't happened, not least because all my friends she's met have been on the left and against the Occupation, but also because, though they keep telling us they're unrepresentative, there does seem to be another Israel, especially among the young. Each family has to face their son's decision to go the army or not, as is the case with Schwebel and his son. His wife Frankie, a music therapist with startling stone-grey eyes, talks about the ongoing psychological damage suffered by many combat soldiers, and for the first of many times, we hear the story of a typical trajectory: do bad things in the army, take off for far-flung places – India, Latin America and increasingly Africa – get stoned for six months to chase out the nightmares, and either come back and re-integrate as a model Israeli husband and father, or don't come back, go into exile.

Schwebel is painting a new series, *A Safe Place*. No longer urban Jerusalem or downtown Tel Aviv, nor haunted by memories of baseball in the Bronx or barbed wire in the camps, these pictures, which we heft out of the studio into the bright daylight, are set in soft-focus landscapes of colour and flowing currents, like a Shakespearean Arcadia, or Prospero's island. A naked man, Schwebel or his double, lies there, no longer the warrior of the streets or the battlefield, but a man seeking rest – like Hanoch Levin's character who cries out for 'some boredom for a change, some Swiss boredom'. The protagonist of these pictures lays his head in the lap of a muse, sometimes more than one muse, at last in a safe place. There's such yearning in these images, such hope and life in Schwebel's irresistible swirls of colour, the forces of nature which no work of men can destroy, hard as they may try.

Hebron

I've been in correspondence with the soldier's peace organisation *Breaking the Silence*. I've asked them to take us to Hebron for the day.

Yehuda, a stocky young man wearing a *kippa*, will be our street-by-street guide to Hebron. As we drive south towards the city, he tells us his story.

'I'm twenty-five, I come from an Orthodox family. I was in the army from 2001 to 2004, based in Hebron. Our job was to protect the settlers.'

They were asked to do things Yehuda thought were wrong. Welding shut people's front doors was the least of it. He went to his commanding officer, and told him he was troubled by his orders.

'Are you refusing to serve?' he said.

'I'm thinking about it.'

He went to see him again. This time he shouted at Yehuda, who replied, 'You don't have the answers, that's why you're yelling.'

He began to realise most Israelis didn't know what was happening in Hebron. He started recording testimonies from soldiers about what they were doing. They made themselves into a group, and called it *Breaking the Silence – Shovrim Shtika*.

In 2004 they decided to put on an exhibition, *Bringing Hebron to Tel Aviv*. Photos, videos, barbed wire, in a photographic gallery in Tel Aviv. More than six thousand people came to the exhibition, from all over the country, many of them soldiers and their families. The gallery became a non-stop talk-in, as soldiers, no longer bearing the burden in silence, were able to tell their families what they had been doing in the occupied territories.

After an hour, we arrive at the outskirts of Hebron – and also the outskirts of the Kiryat Arba settlement, built in 1968 – and walk into a scrubby little park.

'This is the Meir Kahane Memorial Park,' explains Yehuda.

Kahane, a rabbi from Brooklyn, came to Israel, founded an extreme right-wing political party and got himself elected to the Knesset, where he espoused ultra-nationalist laws. We walk into the park, and come to a gravestone, the tomb of Kahane's disciple Baruch Goldstein, who massacred twenty-nine Arabs in a Hebron mosque in 1994. The tomb is still a place of pilgrimage.

We drive into Hebron. And find absolutely nothing and no one in the centre. A void in what used to be a thriving marketplace in front of the venerated Tomb of the Patriarchs, a cathedral-like structure built over the cave where Abraham, a patriarch to Jews, Muslims and Christians, is meant to be buried with his wife Sarah. Other traditions also make it the burial site of Adam and Eve, Isaac and Rebecca and Jacob and Leah.

This city is certainly what philosophers would call 'over-determined'.

Yehuda explains that the army has 'sterilised' the main street. This means that Palestinians are not allowed to walk along it, that their front doors are welded shut and the shopfronts shuttered. Hardly anyone is about. A settler couple scurries past, with their baby. Three souvenir shops are open opposite the Patriarchs' Tomb. The Palestinian shopkeepers greet Yehuda, who has been conducting tours of Hebron for months. A settler with a pistol in his belt drives up with his wife in a jeep and makes uneasy jokes with Yehuda. He has the power to shut the shops.

In what was the meat market, Yehuda points out a solitary Palestinian house next to the walls of one of the town's three settlements. It is draped in wire mesh and netting; the settlers have been stoning it and spitting at it. They also appear to have smashed up a separation wall built between them and Palestinians: chunks of concrete lie around.

Yehuda continues his house-by-house narrative. Jeeps and armoured cars sweep past along the deserted streets opposite the cemetery. Two Arab boys come up and stare at us. Yehuda nervously gets us to move on; they could easily start stoning us.

He reels off case after case where the military administration has given way to the settlers' demands. The whole place is eerily calm, but the walls and the frequent checkpoints seem to exist in the aftermath of violence which could erupt again. Only a few days ago, there was a demonstration against the Annapolis meeting between Arabs and Israelis; two Palestinians were killed. Soldiers run past in jogging gear, rifles slung over their shoulders. Other soldiers, interviewed by *Breaking the Silence*, report attacks on them by settlers who call them Nazis.

I think about the Dizengoff shopping mall back in Tel Aviv. With its busy crowds and piles of merchandise, it's the diametrical opposite of this deserted heart of a city, this *tabula rasa* of occupation. I don't feel like saying much when I return to Tel Aviv and Israeli friends ask what it's been like in Hebron.

Jenin

Juliano Mer Khamis, an actor born in Israel, has stopped acting in order to run the Freedom Theatre of Jenin, a Palestinian town that was the scene of some of the fiercest fighting of the Second Intifada of April 2002. A thousand Israeli combat troops fought some two hundred Palestinians in pitiless house-to-house combat. Civilians were used as human shields. There was looting and theft. Farm land was destroyed. Pornographic graffiti were scrawled on walls.

The Freedom Theatre of Jenin, which Juliano's mother founded, was destroyed. Given the Israel Defence Forces' trashing of arts centres and libraries in other Palestinian cities, and what Elias Khoury calls its determination to inflict cultural and well as ethnic cleansing on Palestinians, there was small chance that a theatre could survive, especially one offering opportunities to young Palestinians, and run by an Israeli who had 'crossed over' to the Enemy.

Juliano, one of Israel's leading actors, has the stature and style of a star: handsome, upright, intense and magnetic. He's as dedicated to this youth theatre as he once was to his career. When he took over the theatre after his mother's death from cancer, he said he wouldn't act in Hebrew again; now he tells me his Arabic isn't good enough to act on the Palestinian stage. If he wants to lead the life of an artist, and not just be a community art therapist, he will have to direct, which he's about to do in Ramallah. Even there he's chosen a confrontational play: *The Lieutenant of Inishmore* by Martin McDonagh, an anti-heroic black comedy about resistance fighters. In Jenin, where every *shahid* (martyr) is idealised on posters hung from lampposts – Hamas and Fatah followers tear down the posters of their political opponents – this play is unlikely to win Juliano a lot of friends.

I met him in London, when he came to show the film he had made about his mother Arna – a strong woman, half-bald from her chemotherapy, seen at the start of the film haranguing Israeli motorists. Arna was an immigrant from Germany, a trained art therapist who came to Palestine in the 'thirties, fought in the *Palmach* against British rule, fell in love with Saliba Khamis, a Palestinian activist, one of the founders of the Israeli Communist Party. She decided to work with Palestinian teenagers to help them dig out and express their anger, frustrations, bitterness and fear. This theatre is not about redemption through art, a lofty alternative to suicide bombing; it's about other ways of existing and resisting, about embattled imagination.

We arrive mid-morning, having driven from the frontier crossing at Kalandia through rolling hills edged with green tufts, valleys surmounted by Jewish settlements commanding a controlling view. After a Palestinian breakfast of falafel and pitta and olives and herbs and dips, Juliano takes us to Jenin's Muslim cemetery, where a large gravestone commemorates the kids from his theatre who died fighting the IDF in 2002. At the entrance to the graveyard someone has spray-painted an Israeli Star of David on the flagstones, obliging visitors to tread on it.

In his two-hundred-seat theatre we watch a succession of young men auditioning to join Juliano's acting classes. They have to do two monologues, a serious one and a comic one, and then sing a song. Only a tiny percentage will be accepted in the classes. The kids are shy, scared to raise their eyes from the floor and stare out into the frightening auditorium. 'This is my favourite bunch,' says Juliano. 'Drug addicts, car thieves, criminals.' This is a leading actor working with them, a perfectionist and a professional – and no stranger to violence within himself; when he played Othello, his Desdemona was so scared of his rage she fled into the wings as he came after her one night.

'Since the Second Intifada,' says Juliano, 'we've run into hostility from local families. They're suspicious of theatre, they think we're going to corrupt their daughters. I have to hold acting classes on separate days for boys and girls. The invasion in 2002 shook people's hope and beliefs. It's the invasion which has caused this retreat into old prejudice and tribal reactions. Every family has an M16 carbine. When we opened, I had to get one of our young men, Zacchariah and his Al Aqsa Brigade boys, to defend our theatre.'

Juliano is scathing about well-meaning Israeli liberals, and about the soul-searching of some refuseniks. 'We shoot and we cry' is the acid way he sums up what he sees as their bad faith. He's lost most of his Israeli friends. He's isolated in this city, rebuilt by the Israeli military with streets wide enough to let tanks and bulldozers through. I was expecting to see the walls pockmarked with bullet-holes, but all the plaster has been made good. Juliano's not optimistic about the future; when I ask him what he expects to be doing in ten years' time, he says, 'Hamas will have taken over. They don't like theatre. They'll throw us from the rooftops.'

I admire the courage and determination of Juliano Mer Khamis. I will try to get theatre friends to visit him and help his theatre. He is laying the foundations for a future Palestinian culture.

Palestinian kids on the streets stare and smile at us, practising their English vocabulary. There's sadness in their eyes. Maybe some of them have lost a brother or a father, in a shoot-out or strapped to a bomb.

Israeli kids have their traumas too. A brother or sister lost in a bus-bomb attack leaves a shaken sister or brother behind.

You see them tumbling out of school in the afternoon, sizzling with energy, kicking a ball, quick as sparrows.

Children are the losers. The scars on both sides will not fade for a long time.

London, December 2007

I come full circle, and in the Gastroenterology Department at University College Hospital, where this story began, I have the colonoscopy I never managed to have in April, when my emergency operation shoved all else aside. Lying on my side, I watch my stomach becoming a television studio, as the consultant pokes a wand with a light and cameras on its end up my arse. It looks like a sequence from one of David Attenborough's wildlife films, without his soothing commentary. Or an underwater documentary by my near-namesake, Jacques Cousteau. Fleshy caverns and tunnels float before the lens, which is searching for signs of malign growth, incipient tumours.

I am given a clean bill of health, and walk warily down to the hospital café, where asparagus soup and rice with meatballs fill my emptied stomach. I'll have another colonoscopy in six months. Meanwhile I keep monitoring my heart, eating carefully and trying to exercise. I guess I'm in remission, or on parole. But then who isn't? We're all born with some calamity in our being; if we're lucky, we can pass a life one step ahead of it.

From David Servan-Schreiber's book *L'Anticancer*, I learn that I'm living out a truce in a total war, no holds barred, against a ruthless enemy. He has a vivid description of the action of cancer cells.

> Attacked by cancer, the organism lives out a total war. Cancerous cells behave like lawless armed gangs, freed from the constraints of the social life which characterise an organism in good health. With their abnormal genes, they are not subject to tissues' mechanisms of regulation. For example, they are not obliged to

die after a certain number of divisions, and therefore become 'immortal'. They turn a deaf ear to signals from surrounding tissues which, alarmed by the lack of space, call on them to stop multiplying. Worse still, they poison them with special substances they secrete. These poisons create an inflammation locally which stimulates their own growth even further, to the detriment of neighbouring territories. Finally, like an army in the field which has to assure its supplies, they requisition adjoining blood vessels and force them to proliferate in order to provide oxygen and nutriments indispensable to the growth of what will rapidly become a tumour.

Cancer is an insurgency.

The metaphors and analogies it prompts are not only with the wars in Iraq and Afghanistan. I have other battlefronts. The house in which I live and work has been hit by an infestation of mice. They gained entry because the house itself is subsiding, and they got in through cracks that have opened in the walls. Urgent action is necessary, say the experts, for the mice breed faster than rabbits, multiplying at insane speed. Like cancer cells.

Rodent operators arrive, lay traps and poison. Contractors assemble, to plan the underpinning of the house. The target part of the property is my garden flat, where these words are being written, where I work every day, where my library has slowly acquired some semblance of order. It's still incomplete, but I have a rough map in my head of where things are, and can usually find whatever I want quickly.

The prospect of the books being heaved into packing cases out of sequence panics me. I had my flat redecorated from top to bottom while I was in hospital, and I returned to it in May with a sense of gratitude that I had a sparkling white-walled haven, a place of quietness and clarity. I got rid of books and hung fewer paintings than I had before, to give the place more stillness. Now all the floors and partition walls will have to come up for the new concrete under-pinning. I'll be out of here for the best part of four months.

Jane says, 'You'll surmount this, the way you've surmounted every-thing else this year.' Maybe; but I anticipate being separated from things I love and need. Needs are immeasurable. I try to calm myself with thoughts about a glass half-empty or half-full and the value of casting things off. But I needed this like a hole in the head.

There's a risk in all writing, and a special risk in this kind of writing.

Most of what I've written in my life has been factual and auto-biographical, analytical or confessional. I'm held in the grip of fact; it's hard for me to envisage fictional transformation of what actually happened. Perhaps only now, writing plays, can I begin to play with my experience.

In the loose form of this personal chronicle, I am trying to cleave to what Stanislavski called 'a through-line', a narrative thread, an intention: I went to India, found I had cancer, was treated, am still recovering – how has it changed me?

I e-mail my therapist, John Witt. He calls back, and we talk for half an hour. 'It's a window into your soul,' he says; I demur at the solemnity of the phrase. 'But why do you want to publish it as a book?' he asks. 'It's so raw the way it is.' I think of the weeks and months of energy, excitement – and yes, narcissism – I have put into it. 'I want to publish it because it seems to me good writing,' I say. I don't say that writing it has kept me going, that I want it out in the world as a sign that *I'm* still in the world. Publishing extracts of it to a mailing list of friends on the internet, which I've done, doesn't fit the bill; it's not really publishing, your text emerges from privacy but doesn't go fully public. Like so much in our lives now, it's a simula-tion of the real thing, a clone of real publication. I want an audience of strangers, of readers I don't know.

I want to leave something behind. Since I have no children, this is what I've made. This is my remnant, my residue, my after-image, my subsequent performance.

I begin and end this book with a death – my mother's in July 2006, and the death of the painter R B Kitaj in October 2007. Writing this book helped keep me going. Getting out of bed at four in the morning and sitting up to write, or scrawling words lying on my back, has been a refusal to let these months slide into oblivion. A refusal, not a refuge. It's also been a quest to find out whether I've changed.

At first I resisted wrapping up what I've written in a tidy summation or coda. Resolution, knitting threads and tying up ends, seems alien to what I feel now. But if it can't be a full-company walk-down finale, it's nonetheless a terminus.

I think of myself less like a *juvens,* more a *senex*; less juvenile, not yet senile; able to play the senior-actor lead roles in my life, leaving the splashy, showy, dashing parts to the juvenile leads. Less the son-child, battering at the supremacy of fathers and father-figures or buttering up to their power. More aware of how much political rage is stoked by displaced Oedipal stuff, spilt psychology.

I've become both less of a Jew and more Jewish. Over the eighteen months I've described here, with their associative loops and flash-backs, I can see the shift from my unthinking adherence to my native Jewish tribe to my abandonment of inherited attitudes and reflexes, to a position of neither obedience nor childish defiance.

I've learned – not least from Jane, her quick and immediate political reflexes – to use my anger, to lay about me rather than lie about and on myself. During this passage from India there have been many reasons to be depressed. Yet I've been downcast, flummoxed, set back, but so far never trapped in the quagmire of depression. Anger, indignation, scorn have helped me keep at bay the Churchillian 'black dog'. At the same time – again, tutored by Jane's example, the way she uses the adjective 'sweet' to celebrate all manner of people – I've expressed simpler, less sentimental love for others. Life's just more interesting when you do.

Becoming the most minimal sort of grandfather to Jane's grandsons – an underperforming grandad, wary still of venturing out of my solitude, where I am in control, into family, where I'm at sea – has nonetheless loosened some of my armour-plating. But I still put limits on the amount of play, of child's play, I can allow myself.

March 2008

Paul Scofield dies, of leukaemia, in Sussex, aged 86.

In one of the obituaries, he's quoted as saying that he'd got so used to being described by journalists as a private person that 'I half-expect people to phone me and say, "Hello, is that Paul Scofield, the very private person?"'

He was Peter Brook's creative double and his mirror, his elective affinity. In my Brook biography I wrote of their formative impact on each other as young men at Birmingham Rep in 1946. I'd written to Scofield asking him to write about working with Brook, and he replied in two short letters, clearly painful to write.

'We were different from each other,' Scofield noted, 'I a few years older and an actor, he an intellectual who was also an artist. I remember that I felt that for him an actor was not very interesting.'

As they worked, on Shaw's *Man and Superman*, Shakespeare's *King John* and *Love's Labours Lost*, Scofield taught Brook as well as learning from him. 'There was a change,' he wrote of Brook;

> Perhaps the daily experience of working with a company of actors and actresses in developing his interpretations of the plays, as opposed to following a pre-prepared scheme of action, fundamentally altered his vision.

Scofield remained a tacit, even a shy man, and an immense, mischievous and mysterious actor.

Page proofs arrive for *The Half*, Simon Annand's big book of photographs of actors in their dressing rooms preparing to go on stage, for which I've written an introduction. As well as a being a fresco of twenty-five years of theatre, it's also a document of the inhospitable and unwelcoming conditions of most dressing-rooms. Sunk below ground level, and without a toilet, actors' quarters were like cattle boxes.

Looking at Simon's photographs for *The Half*, I am reminded of Hamlet's speech when he finds Yorick's skull in the graveyard. 'Where be your gibes now? your gambols? your songs? your flashes of merriment, that were wont to set the table on a roar? Not one now, to mock your own grinning?'

Acting alters space and time, and makes a stand against time's erasure. To act is to defy oblivion. In the end, all actors can rely on is their audience's memories.

Simon's photographs scrupulously and steadily observe actors in the changing room, the room of change, getting ready for the night's work in a profession of transience.

Palestinian rockets are hitting Israeli towns. Israel retaliates massively with satellite-guided air-strikes on the Gaza refugee camps.

> SatNav / that's the way to do it
> Get them in your sights / at 30,000 feet
> Kick in a stick of shiny missiles
> Punch a row of holes in the houses on the street
>
> Moshe, commander, orders up an air-strike
> Sends it from his base at company HQ
> to Avram, pilot, his ace missile launcher
> Avram will know what he has to do

Laila, civilian, and her kids are watching telly
Celebrity Big Brother in Arabic
Volume too high, and there isn't a siren
Big mistake / when your walls aren't thick

SatNav / everybody's watching
Satellite surveillance 24-7
Put a foot wrong and Big Brother knows it
Cut the wrong profile and you land in Heaven

Mahmoud launches / a home-made rocket
Thrusts across the Negev to doomed Sderot
Sderot homes haven't got SatNav
Only twenty seconds before it hits the spot

Avram watches, then presses his button
Missiles of Murder / Angels of Death
Wing their way down to enemy targets
Taking out their houses, sucking out their breath

Avram, satisfied, shoots his load
Checks he has scored an accurate hit
Bombing reminds him of dropping a turd
To add to the mounting bucket of shit

they are making of Gaza. Mission complete
Autoguide SatNav / ensures he'll get back
Ready for orders in his cockpit seat
Permanently ready, always on track

SatNav SatNav / keeps the world spinning
Give us our SatNav / wait for the thud
SatNav SatNav / nobody's winning
Everyone's swimming in a sea of blood
SatNav SatNav / nobody's grinning
SatNav primed and ready to send

Everyone knows this is just a beginning
SatNav SatNav where will it end?

The comparison of bombs with turds comes from my daily familiarity with the colostomy bag I am wearing on my stomach, to keep the surgery wound from being infected. I've been wearing it for a year, and have got better at aiming turds into the bowl, hence the image of the blitz as shit. Next month I go back to hospital for an operation to remove the bag and tie up loose ends.

I don't believe in cultural boycotts. Writing, and the arts as a whole, should not be used as instruments of coercion. Art is there to embody and remind us of our common humanity. On the wall of my lobby I have hung a sprightly handbill, printed in old woodblock lettering and published by an American theatre group, the Bread and Puppet Theatre. They gave it to me after I brought them to London with their anti-Vietnam War play *Fire*. I look at it once or twice a day as I go in and out. It's a kind of secular *mezuzah*.

Ancestral Jewish joke.

A Jew in midlife comes to realise that he can't take it any more, all this Jewishness, this hatred and strife and history and feverish debate, all this effort, all these loud voices in his head and around him when he goes to *shul*.

He decides to convert, and becomes a Catholic.

He's very serious about it, studies the lives of the saints, goes to confession, participates in requiems for the dead.

Years pass.

One Sunday at church, they come to him and say, 'You are such a perfect Christian, we'd like to offer you an honour. Preach the sermon next Sunday.'

The man says, 'No I couldn't. I'm only a convert, it wouldn't be right.'

the WHY CHEAP ART? manifesto

PEOPLE have been THINKING too long that
ART is a PRIVILEGE of the MUSEUMS & the
RICH. ART IS NOT BUSINESS !
It does not belong to banks & fancy investors
ART IS FOOD . You cant EAT it BUT it FEEDS
you . ART has to be CHEAP & available to
EVERYBODY . It needs to be EVERYWHERE
because it is the INSIDE of the
WORLD .

ART SOOTHES PAIN !
Art wakes up sleepers !
ART FIGHTS AGAINST WAR & STUPIDITY !
ART SINGS HALLELUJA !
ART IS FOR KITCHENS !
ART IS LIKE GOOD BREAD!
Art is like green trees !
Art is like white clouds in blue sky !
ART IS CHEAP !
HURRAH
Bread & Puppet Glover, Vermont. 1984

'We insist,' they reply; 'you are a credit to our congregation. You must give the sermon. '

They persuade him.

Next Sunday, he mounts the pulpit. He looks round the church. It is packed with expectant, well-wishing friends.

His heart swells. He opens his arms, and raises his voice and begins, 'My fellow Jews....'

I go to a requiem for Suzanne Goodwin, wife of John Goodwin, my first boss and comrade in the theatre. Suzanne died at the age of 92. She was a bustling, bright woman who wrote a stream of romantic novels. She was a Catholic, and the requiem, the first I've ever been to, is in a church in Hammersmith, with a poor, rather sad, congregation who seem to have turned out for the ceremony because it's better than staying at home.

I stand in a side aisle, watch John, standing in front of the basket-work coffin, still a dapper, curly-haired, boyish figure. He gave me my first lessons in typography, printing and design, when I went to work for him at Stratford upon Avon in 1962 to create the illustrated theatre programmes for the Royal Shakespeare Company. He had an infectious giggle and was a stern editor, wielding an elegant propelling pencil over what he called my 'lapel-grabbing prose'. He was the first person I met who owned a retractable champagne swizzle stick. He and Suzanne had a lot of style of a certain English class and period; they reminded me of characters in an Anthony Powell novel.

In a tribute, Suzanne's niece reads from a letter about Suzanne from a young woman: 'Suzanne taught me how to make salad dressing and mend a broken heart.'

Meanwhile, I've been neglecting my play. As Kops keeps reminding me. He never stops wanting me to take a deep breath and move away from my old self into a new one. I meant to make a fresh start on a much-changed new draft of the play a month ago, but things intervened. Or I cooked up things to do that stopped me getting back into the flow if writing it.

For weeks I have left my principal character holed up in a dusty cafe in Gaza City, with shells falling and machine-gun fire in the street outside.

I tinker with his monologue:

What the fuck, to quote my son, am I doing here? Fuck knows. I came to dig up fragments of history. And I find myself *in* history, dodging bullets in a battlefield.

Yesterday, from my hidey-hole I saw something totally bloody awful, even by the standards of this place.

A man, forties, is on his knees, weeping his heart out over the corpse of a teenage boy. He's rocking to get the grief out, he's banging his head with his fists, he's wailing like an old woman, you've seen it on the screen.

Eventually he gets up, bends to pick up the boy. Round the corner comes a gunman. Balaclava, shades, Kalashnikov. 'Stop!' he shouts at the man. 'Stay where you are!'

'But I have to bury my son,' says the man. 'I have to cover him with earth. It's respect for the dead.'

'I know your face,' says the gunman. 'You're Fatah. Fucking Fatah. Leave the boy where he is. No burial, no grave. The boy's ours now. We'll parade him in a funeral for the cameras. Just fuck off out of here, my friend, or I'll blow your head off. Understand?'

In the Trojan War, they tied Hector's corpse to a chariot and dragged him through the city. They needed to dismember the hero. To mutilate hope. But this is worse.

When I get back to it, all this may go out of the window.

I must get to the end of this draft in the next three weeks, before I go into hospital to have my bowel operation reversed. I remember the good resolutions of the narrator of Italo Svevo's *La coscienza di Zeno*. The first chapter begins with the words, 'Today I smoked my last cigarette'. So do the following chapters. It's one of literature's best running gags.

I'm still straddling the same dichotomy: am I a producer who writes, or a writer who produces? A maker of books, essays, plays, or a purveyor of shows, programmes and films? What is my real identity?

Do I have to have only one? If I diffuse myself in deeds, is that a subtraction, a distraction, from writing? Or does it feed writing?

For all his warmth, Kops gets incensed with my detours and alibis: 'Do you want to be remembered as a good producer of other people's talent, or do you want to take your own talent seriously?'

I go back to hospital. The operation to reconnect my innards works. I begin to dream about sitting in my garden.

Then, three days after the operation, I have a heart arrest.

Take it from Me

I am talking
to Jane I think
but I could be wrong
in bed in this room
full of colours

Then I can hear nothing
and
a
blind

begins to come down
leeching all colours

turning everything blue

This blue blind descends steadily
sucking up all colour all sound

This is an ending
A sharks' tooth bares
to snatch me down

They shock my heart back on track
but I have seen it now
this sneak preview of my death

Saturday, May 24, 2008

Dear friends and loved ones,

After thirty-five days in hospital, days of mind-numbing tedium, void and occasional fear, I am home. I have a new bedfellow, a defibrillator or pacemaker, under my chest skin. She is devoted to my heart, and steadies it.

Now I know a little more about my heart arrest, I realise what great luck I have had. If the person in bed opposite me had not seen me slump and drop my book; if it all hadn't happened in hospital but outside, I could have lost time, brain cells, and maybe had speech affected. As it was, I had 66 electric shocks before my heart was put back on track.

Our lives hang by such threads.

Parade

Down the street you snake your way
Kerb to kerb, earth to sky
Holding aloft on a fragile rod
A placard with letters drawn in blood
Slogans running in the rain
Battered backpacks heavy with pain
Marching for change, marching for good
  The multitude

Open coffins draped with flags
Zipped-up unmarked body bags
Tipped into pits, burned on pyres
Liquefied in holy fires
Martyr and murderer, mother and child
Scraps of child-flesh scattered in the dust
If the rockets don't get you, the bus-bombers must
  Sad multitude

Kitaj the Jewish painter's gone
Glittering-fingered Peterson
Impish actor Normington
The famous the finest the fabled the phoney
Bergman and Antonioni
Dark dark they've all gone into the dark
Latecomers in the deserted park
Swallowed by the hungry wood
  Lost multitude

And yet the flood of people moves on
Stumbling over the dead and the gone
Tumbling, staggering, arriving, leaving
Weeping, leaping, laughing, grieving
Your destiny perpetual motion
Parading itself your destination
Dreams are your drink, hoping your food
  Never-ending multitude

Angelus Novus painted by Klee
Backing forwards, turning away
From the garbage heap of history
The past a demolished disaster zone
Playgrounds rubble, shattered homes
The ground is burning under our feet
Get out of the way if you can't stand the heat
Don't abandon the march, it's your only chance
If you can't go on walking, learn to dance
If the best is impossible, settle for the good
  O multitude

May 2008

A SELECTION OF BOOKS

David Servan-Schreiber, *L'Anticancer* (Robert Laffont: Paris, 2007)

Philip Roth, *The Facts* (Jonathan Cape: London, 1981)

R B Kitaj, *Second Diasporist Manifesto* (Oxford University Press: Oxford, 2007)

Bertolt Brecht, *Poems* (Methuen: London, 1976)

Harold Pinter, *The Homecoming* (Faber and Faber: London, 1991)

Bernard Kops, *The World is a Wedding* (McGibbon & Kee: London, 1967)

Bernard Kops, *Shalom Bomb* (Oberon Books, London: 2000)

Franz Kafka, *Works and Texts* (Penguin: Harmondsworth, 1976)

Arnold Wesker, *All Things Tire of Themselves* (Flambard Press: Newcastle upon Tyne, 2008)

Isaac Deutscher, *The Non-Jewish Jew and other Essays* (Oxford University Press; Oxford, 1968)

Ian Nairn, *Nairn's Paris* (Penguin: Harmondsworth, 1971)

Eyal Weizman, *Hollow Land: Israel's Architecture of Occupation* (Verso: London, 2007)